Cardiopulmonary Pharmacology

A Handbook for Respiratory Practitioners and Other Allied Health Personnel

Cardiopulmonary Pharmacology

A Handbook for Respiratory Practitioners and Other Allied Health Personnel

Cynthia L. Howder, R.R.T., C.P.F.T.

Acting Program Director/Instructor
Respiratory Therapy Program
Seattle Central Community College
Seattle, Washington
Instructor
Respiratory Therapy Program
Tacoma Community College
Tacoma, Washington

WILLIAMS & WILKINS
BALTIMORE • HONG KONG • LONDON • MUNICH
PHILADELPHIA • SYDNEY • TOKYO

Editor: John P. Butler
Managing Editor: Linda Napora
Copy Editor: Thomas Lehr
Designer: Karen S. Klinedinst
Illustration Planner: Wayne Hubbel
Production Coordinator: Anne Stewart Seitz

Printed in the United States of America

Library of Congress Cataloging-in-Publication Data

Howder, Cynthia L.
Cardiopulmonary pharmacology : a handbook for respiratory practitioners and other allied health personnel / Cynthia L. Howder.
p. cm.
Includes bibliographical references and index.
ISBN 0-683-04175-4
1. Pulmonary pharmacology—Handbooks, manuals, etc. 2. Cardiopulmonary system—Effect of drugs on—Handbooks, manuals, etc. 3. Respiratory therapists. I. Title.
[DNLM: 1. Allied Health Personnel. 2. Heart Diseases—drug therapy. 3. Respiratory Tract Diseases—drug therapy. WF 145 H854c]
RM388.H68 1992
616.1'2061—dc20
DNLM/DLC
for Library of Congress 91-10345
CIP

91 92 93 94 95
1 2 3 4 5 6 7 8 9 10

Affectionately dedicated to my two best friends,
Steve and Brenda

Preface

The primary purpose of *Cardiopulmonary Pharmacology* is to familiarize the respiratory practitioner, the student, and other allied health personnel with the most commonly used cardiopulmonary drugs. Also presented are drugs used in cardiac arrest and drugs commonly given to the critically ill patient.

In Section I, the first six chapters introduce the reader to drug therapy: principles and administration, phases of pharmacologic action and effect, drug interactions and modifications, evaluation, dosages and calculations, and drug preparation.

In Section II, the major portion of this handbook, Chapters 7 through 20 present the individual pharmacologic agents with criteria for use, administration, actions and effects, contraindications, and adverse effects. Also, when necessary, a brief review of basic physiology and anatomy is included to help the learner fully understand how a particular drug or drug type affects the body.

To enhance the learner's awareness, each chapter has a list of objectives, emphasizing the primary points and goals of the chapter.

A comprehensive assessment test (at the end of this book) closely follows in format (multiple choice, true-false, clinical simulations) the national examinations taken by practitioners. This test will be particularly helpful in preparing for the examinations.

Cynthia L. Howder, R.R.T., C.P.F.T.

Acknowledgments

A very sincere and special thank you to the following for their support, encouragement, and advice:

John Butler, Executive Editor, and
John Gardner, Vice President and Publisher, Williams & Wilkins

Mike Cline, R.R.T., Instructor, Respiratory Therapy Program,
Tacoma Community College, Tacoma, Washington

Brenda Connors, R.N., Orthopedic Charge Nurse,
St. Joseph's Hospital, Tacoma, Washington

Contents

Introduction to Drug Therapy

I

General Principles of Pharmacology 1

Comprehending drugs and their actions and effects is the basis of pharmacology. All drugs alter or enhance the body's own natural system through biochemical and physiological effects. The dose of a drug and the selectivity of a drug's effect is of special importance and a major consideration in therapeutics. Pharmacology is unique not only because it plays a significant part in medicine but also because it deals substantially with the mechanisms of action of biologically active substances.

Objectives

1. Specify the five types of drug sources and give an example of each.
2. List and define the five types of drug names.
3. Name the official publication for drug standards.
4. Identify the major sources for drug information.
5. Discuss the legal factors involved with drugs.
6. Explain the major parts of the written prescription.
7. Define the pharmacological terms presented.
8. Associate a standard abbreviation with its meaning.

Drug Sources

Drugs originate from five major sources:

Animal sources—Examples include thyroxin (a purified compound obtained from the thyroid gland of an animal), used for the treatment of hypothyroidism, and insulin (obtained from the pancreata of hogs, sheep, and cattle), used in the treatment of diabetes mellitus.

Vegetable or plant sources—Examples include digitalis, which originates from the dried leaves of the purple foxglove plant, used in the treatment of congestive heart failure and cardiac arrhythmias. Atropine and scopolamine are obtained from the plant *Atropa belladonna.* Also, morphine sulfate, cocaine, nicotine, and caffeine all originate from parts of plants.

Mineral sources—These drugs are usually formed from acids, bases, and salts found in food. Calcium, potassium chloride, copper sulfate, and magnesium sulfate originate from mineral sources.

Synthetic sources—The most common source of drugs today. This group is composed of compounds formed from the natural elements. Examples include the synthetic steroids and sulfonamides.

Genetic engineering—This relatively new and exciting source of drugs has opened a new concept to pharmacology. The most recent advances include the cloning and production of human insulin and tissue plasminogen activator (TPA). TPA is the newest thrombolytic agent used to treat myocardial infarction (see also Chapter 20). Initially, TPA was isolated from blood, various tissues, and blood vessels. Yet the amounts that could be purified were not enough for any extensive use. TPA is now produced through genetically engineered cells in culture.

DRUG NAMES

Official name—issued to the drug by the official pharmaceutical publications.

Code name—issued to the drug while in the development or research phase.

Generic name—issued to the drug by the company developing the drug. Sometimes the same as the official name.

Chemical name—the drug's structural formula.

Proprietary name (brand or trade name)—issued to the drug by the legal owner or manufacturer of the drug.

Example: Albuterol
Official name: albuterol
Generic name: albuterol (international generic name: salbutamol)
Chemical name: (α^1-[(*tert*-butylamino)methyl]-4-hydroxy-*m*-xylene-α,α'-diol)
Proprietary names: Proventil, Ventolin

DRUG STANDARDS

The *United States Pharmacopeia* (USP) is an authoritative book that sets forth drug standards to ensure uniformity of strength for drugs and standards for identification and purity of drugs. Drugs listed in this pharmacopeia are official drugs that legally conform to the standards and are marked "USP."

The *National Formulary* (NF) is sponsored by the American Pharmaceutical Association and contains formulas for drug mixtures or single drugs. Since 1980 the USP and NF have been consolidated into a single volume.

SOURCES FOR DRUG INFORMATION

United States Dispensatory: This is an encyclopedia that contains survey articles and detailed accounts on individual drugs. Official, nonproprietary, trade, and chemical names of drugs are given along with monographs that contain histories, descriptions, actions, uses, facts on toxicology, and doses of drugs.

AMA Drug Evaluations: This publication details current drugs and also new drugs that have not yet been included in the USP. This book is useful in describing accepted therapeutic practices.

Physicians' Desk Reference (PDR): The PDR contains an annual listing of drugs from various manufacturers. The volume is arranged in five sections, including a section containing full-size color photographs of various capsules and tablets. It gives useful information of brand name products and a list of manufacturers with their products. Also included is information on action, uses, administration, dosage, contraindications, and composition of each drug.

Drug Facts and Comparisons: Composed by various pharmacists and doctors, this book provides a broad range of drug information.

Goodman and Gilman's *The Pharmacological Basis of Therapeutics:* This book gives in-depth detail to each facet of pharmacology and makes an excellent source for study.

DRUG LEGISLATION

Twentieth-century drug therapy has seen some remarkable changes that affect the control, distribution, and use of drugs. Among these are the improvement and promotion of legislation regarding the sale and manufacture of drugs. Some of the more important acts of legislation regarding the manufacture and sale of drugs are:

- The U.S. Food and Drug Acts of 1906 (USP and NF were given official status), 1938 (Food, Drug and Cosmetic Act became law), and 1962 (Kefauver-Harris Law passed requiring the proof of safety and efficacy of all drugs introduced since 1938).

- The Harrison Narcotic Act of 1914 (governs the sale and distribution of all narcotics).
- The Controlled Substance Act of 1971. In 1971 the federal government imposed further restrictions on prescription drugs that have a high potential for abuse:

Class I—potential for abuse is high. These drugs have no accepted medical use and lack accepted safety as drugs. Examples are heroin, LSD, PCP, marihuana, and methaqualone.

Class II—potential for abuse is high. These drugs have accepted medical use with severe restrictions. Abuse may lead to psychologic or physical dependence. These prescriptions cannot be refilled. Examples are narcotics (opium, codeine, morphine, etc.), stimulants (cocaine, amphetamine), and depressants (amobarbital, pentobarbital, secobarbital).

Class III—potential for abuse is less than that of drugs in class I or II. These drugs have accepted current medical use. They have moderate to low potential for physical dependence and high potential for psychologic dependence. There is a 5-refill maximum with no refill available after 6 months from the date of the initial order. Examples are codeine combinations, glutethimide, and phendimetrazine.

Class IV—potential for abuse is less than class III drugs. These drugs have accepted current medical use and a limited potential for dependence. Examples are diazepam, flurazepam, phentermine, and propoxyphene.

Class V—potential for abuse is less than class IV drugs. These drugs have current accepted medical use and potential for dependence is low. These agents may be dispensed without a prescription unless state regulations apply. Examples are cold and cough preparations with codeine and diphenoxylate combinations (Lomotil is prescription only).

LEGAL FACTORS

There are two recognized classes of drugs: over-the-counter (OTC) drugs and drugs that require a prescription from a physician. OTC drugs require no prescription and may be safely self-administered by the lay person. Approximately 50% of all drug doses are OTC.

Prescription drugs are controlled by the U.S. Food and Drug Administration. They can be identified by the statement: "Caution: Federal law prohibits dispensing without a prescription." All prescription drugs require this statement, as well as a package insert. The package brochure lists the indications, contraindications, warnings, and dosing regimen for the drug.

PRESCRIPTION WRITING

A prescription is an order for medication written by a physician (Fig. 1.1). The drug may be prescribed by its official name, by its nonproprietary name (also called generic name), or by a manufacturer's trade name.

In the hospital setting, medications are prescribed in the patient's chart on a particular page (usually the physician's order pages). This type of prescription order is known as a chart order. The contents usually include the name and strength of the drug, the dose, the route and frequency of administration, the date, and the prescriber's signature.

The contents of a hospital chart order and an outpatient prescription are similar. Normally, an outpatient prescription is written in a certain order and consists of four primary parts:

Superscription—This is simply Rx (the abbreviation for "recipe," meaning take thou).

Inscription—This indicates the drug's ingredients and its amounts. If a drug contains several ingredients, it is customary to list the principal ingredient first.

Subscription—This contains the directions for dispensing.

Signature—Usually abbreviated as "sig," this contains instructions for the patient, such as "take one teaspoonful four times daily."

Bill Leffler, M.D.
523 S. Prairie Avenue
City
Telephone: 362-8953

NAME Paul Thackara **AGE** 40
ADDRESS 3214 N. G St. **DATE** 3/12/90

(1) ℞ (2) Tetracycline, 250 mg capsules
(3) Dispense 20
Repeat ☐ (4) Label: Take one capsule four times daily
Nonrepeat ☒
D.E.A. No. ______

______ M.D. ______ M.D.
Generic Substitution Permitted Dispense as Written

Figure 1.1. The typical prescription. 1, Superscription; 2, inscription; 3, subscription; 4, signature. See text for explanation.

In addition to these four parts, the prescription should have the patient's name and the physician's signature followed by the prescriber's degree.

GLOSSARY OF TERMS

acetylcholinesterase (AChE)—An enzyme that destroys acetylcholine.

acetyltransferase—Enzymes that have the ability to catalyze the transfer of an acetyl group from one entity to another (e.g., choline acetyltransferase is an enzyme that brings about the synthesis of acetylcholine).

acidosis—A pathological condition in the body resulting from an accumulation of acid or from reduced amounts of base.

adrenergic—Epinephrine-like effects; the nerve fibers activated by norepinephrine or epinephrine or any agent that produces such an effect.

adrenergic receptor (adrenoceptor)—Innervated by postganglionic adrenergic fibers. In the sympathetic system, these receptors are classified as α-adrenergic and β-adrenergic receptors.

agonist—Drug affinity to a specific receptor site. The drug has the ability to produce an effect.

alkalosis—A pathological condition in the body resulting in excessive alkalinity owing to a loss of acid or an accumulation of base.

analeptic—Medication to restore consciousness or alertness (i.e., doxapram, caffeine).

analgesic—Medication to relieve pain (aspirin, morphine) without causing loss of consciousness.

anaphylaxis—An exaggerated or unusual reaction of an organism to a foreign substance. The resultant reaction may be life threatening.

anesthetic—Medication causing a loss of sensation.

antagonist—Drug affinity to a specific receptor site. The drug does not produce a physiological effect itself. The drug blocks the action and effect of an agonist.

antiadrenergic—Blocking an adrenergic response.

antibiotics—Medication used to kill microorganisms that cause infectious diseases.

antibodies—Substances within the body that react with a specific antigen; abbreviated Ab.

anticholinesterase (anti-AChE)—Any drug that has the ability to inhibit the enzyme acetylcholinesterase, thereby potentiating the effects of acetylcholine at the postsynaptic receptor site.

antigen—Any substance that leads to the development of antibodies, inducing a specific immune response. Abbreviated Ag.

autocoid—Various endogenous substances that do not yet fit into a functional classification (histamine, serotonin, prostaglandins).

autonomic—Capable of self function; self-governing.

bioavailability—The rate at which a drug becomes available to a receptor after its administration; gives an estimate of how much of a drug's dose is effective.

blocker—Any agent that has the ability to inhibit a neurotransmitter's action at the effector organ.

catalyst—A substance that has the ability to increase the reaction of a chemical process, but itself is not consumed in the reaction.

catecholamines—A group of sympathomimetic amines (neurohormones) produced by the adrenal medulla and adrenergic nerve endings that cause an adrenergic response on the autonomic nervous system. Examples are dopamine, epinephrine, and norepinephrine.

cholinergic—Acetylcholine-like effects; the nerve fibers activated by acetylcholine or any agent that produces such an effect.

cholinergic receptor (cholinoceptor)—Innervated by cholinergic nerve fibers located at both the sympathetic and parasympathetic ganglionic synapses. Also, the postganglionic nerve fibers of the parasympathetic system (muscarinic) and the neuromuscular junction of skeletal muscles (nicotinic).

conjugation—The merging of a toxic substance with an endogenous natural substance to form a detoxified product.

degradation—Making a chemical compound less complex by separating one or more groups of its atoms.

degranulation—The breaking up of a substance into smaller particles (e.g., the splitting open of the mast cell).

diuretic—A medication that increases urine flow.

dosage—The regulation of the frequency and number of doses.

dose—The quantity of a drug to be given to a patient at one time.

drug efficacy—A drug's ability to utilize its effect and activate a receptor site.

drug potency—The amount of dose required to produce an effect.

facilitative—A reaction produced as an indirect result of a drug's action (e.g., an infection resulting from altering the natural flora of the body by administering antibiotics).

glycogenolysis—A reaction produced in the liver where glucose is formed from the splitting up of glycogen.

half-life—The length of time it takes for an amount of drug to be reduced by half within the body.

hypertonic solution—Having greater osmotic pressure than the mixture with which it is compared.

hypotonic solution—Having less osmotic pressure than the mixture with which it is compared.

iatrogenic—An adverse reaction resulting from treatment given by a physician.

idiosyncrasy—Exaggerated reaction to drugs; unusual susceptibility to a drug or substance.

isotonic solution—Having the same osmotic pressure as the mixture with which it is compared.

kinins—Peptides that cause increased vascular permeability, induce hypotension, and cause contraction of smooth muscle.

mediator—A substance that has the ability to affect a process or produce a reaction.

narcotic—Medication that produces stupor or sleep and relieves pain.

pharmacodynamics—The physiological mechanism of action of drugs and their biochemical effects.

pharmacokinetics—The movement of a drug within the body over a period of time. Includes the processes of absorption, distribution, biotransformation, and excretion.

pharmacotherapeutics—The study of the prevention and treatment of disease states with drugs and medications.

phosphodiesterase—An enzyme that inactivates the cAMP system.

stimulus—Any agent that produces a reaction in a receptor.

STANDARD ABBREVIATIONS

aa	of each	Cu	copper
ac	before meals	d	day
ad	to, up to	DNR	do not resuscitate
ad lib	as much as desired	et	and
alt hor	every other hour	ex aq	in water
bid	twice daily	°F	Fahrenheit
c̄	with	Fe	iron
°C	Celsius	fl	fluid
cal	calorie	g, gm	gram
cc	cubic centimeter	gal	gallon
Cl	chloride	gr	grain
cu	cubic	gtt	drop

h	hour
hs	bedtime
I	iodine
IM	intramuscular
IU	international unit
IV	intravenous
I & O	intake and output
K	potassium
kg	kilogram
L, l	liter
lb	pound
m	meter
mcg, μg	microgram
mEq	milliequivalent
mg	milligram
Mg	magnesium
ml	milliliter
mm	millimeter
Na	sodium
NF	National Formulary
non rep	not to be repeated
NPO	nothing by mouth
od	right eye
os	left eye
otc	over the counter
oz	ounce
P	phosphorus
pc	after meals
po	by mouth
prn	as needed
pro rect	rectally
pt	pint
pulv	powder
q	every
qd	every day
qh	every hour
qid	four times daily
qod	every other day
qs	as much as needed
qt	quart
Rx	prescription only
s̄	without
s̄s̄	one-half
SC	subcutaneous
sig	write
sol	solution
stat	immediately
tab	tablet
t½	half-life
tid	three times daily
tbsp, T	tablespoon
tsp	teaspoon
U	unit
UD	unit dose
ung	ointment
Zn	zinc

ʒ	dram
♏	minim
oz or ℥	ounce
℈	scruple
μ	micro

2 Divisions of and Actions within the Autonomic Nervous System

Since the site for pharmacological manipulation of cardiopulmonary drugs is the autonomic nervous system, familiarity with its system and activities is essential.

Objectives

1. Define the terms neuron, soma, axon, dendrite, synapse, synaptic junction.
2. Classify the two primary types of neurotransmitters and give examples of each.
3. Explain the major tasks and functions of the autonomic nervous system.
4. Identify the organs innervated by the sympathetic system and the parasympathetic system. State which system, the sympathetic or the parasympathetic, dominates under stressful situations.
5. Define efferent, ganglion, preganglionic neuron, postganglionic neuron.
6. List the neurotransmitters of the ANS. State where each neurotransmitter is stored and describe the effects each has on the sympathetic and parasympathetic systems.
7. Discuss the synthesis, storage, and release of norepinephrine and acetylcholine.
8. Explain the autonomic receptor theory. Also explain adrenergic receptor and cholinergic receptor. Identify the actions and effects produced when an adrenergic receptor is stimulated and when a cholinergic receptor is stimulated.
9. Describe the effects COMT, MAO have on catecholamines.

10. Differentiate between muscarinic and nicotinic effects as related to acetylcholine.
11. Define competitive inhibition and give an example.
12. Explain adrenergic drug action and discuss the process that occurs when an adrenergic receptor is stimulated.
13. Define cAMP, phosphodiesterase, catecholamine, indirect acting sympathomimetic, direct acting sympathomimetic.
14. Explain antiadrenergic drug action.
15. Describe the effects α blocking agents, β blocking agents have on adrenergic receptors.
16. Discuss cholinergic drug action and the process that occurs when a cholinergic receptor is stimulated.
17. Define cGMP, acetylcholinesterase, direct acting parasympathomimetic, indirect acting parasympathomimetic.
18. Explain anticholinergic drug action.
19. List the primary and secondary effects a cholinergic blocking agent produces in respect to the body's respiratory system.
20. Identify and discuss the various mediators that affect bronchomotor tone.

REVIEW OF NEURONS, SYNAPSES, AND NEUROTRANSMITTERS

Nervous tissue is the fundamental element of the nervous system and consists of two cell types: neurons (nerve cells that direct impulses to and from all parts of the body) and neuroglia (supporting and protecting cells to the neuron). Each neuron (Fig. 2.1) consists of a nerve cell body (soma) and nerve fibers (one axon and one or more dendrites). An axon extends from the nerve cell body and conducts impulses away from (efferent) the cell body. Dendrites are generally shorter than axons and serve to conduct impulses toward (afferent) the cell body.

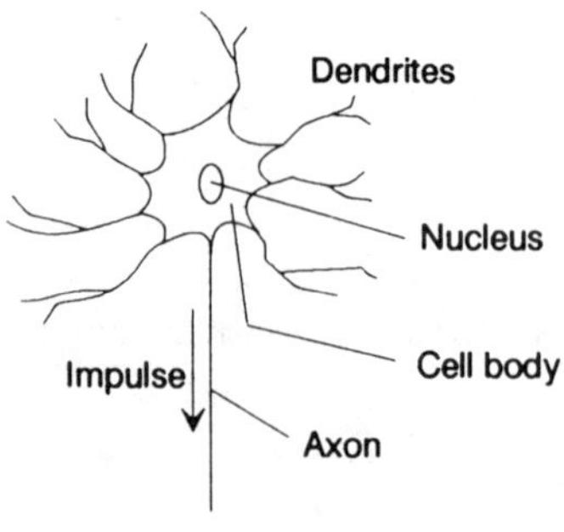

Figure 2.1. The neuron.

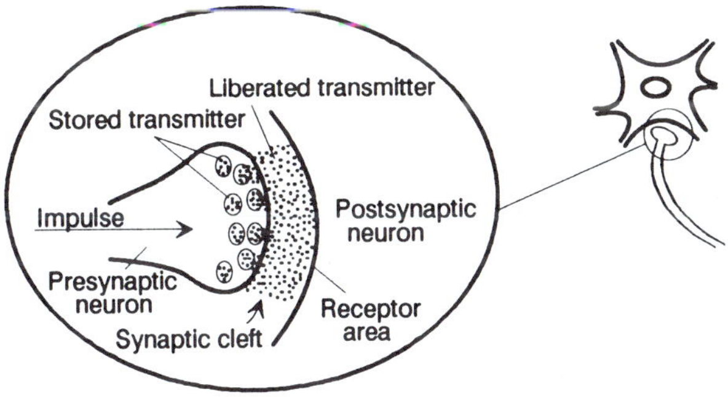

Figure 2.2. The synaptic junction.

Since each neuron is separate in and of itself, a synaptic junction exists between neurons (Fig. 2.2). The synapse controls the passage and direction of impulses through neurotransmitter chemicals. The neurotransmitter chemical is stored in the axon terminals of a neuron. When an impulse is generated, the neurotransmitter substance is liberated from the presynaptic neuron into the synaptic cleft. A transient change in the membrane permeability of the postsynaptic neuron is generated, allowing the neurotransmitter to bind to a receptor on the postsynaptic cell membrane. Neurotransmitter action is rapidly aborted by one or more medians: (*a*) enzymatic metabolism of the neurotransmitter by the effector organ; (*b*) enzymatic degradation of the neurotransmitter in the synaptic cleft; (*c*) if reuptake of the neurotransmitter into the presynaptic neuron occurs, it may be degraded by an enzyme there; or (*d*) the neurotransmitter may be taken back into the storage site. Also, a small amount is carried away in the blood.

Two types of neurotransmitter substances have been documented. Those that cause excitation (such as norepinephrine, acetylcholine, dopamine, histamine, and serotonin) and those that cause inhibition (such as glycine and γ-aminobutyric acid [GABA]). Synapses are sensitive to pH, a lack of oxygen, fatigue, and drugs. When these factors are present the relay of impulses may be affected.

CENTRAL AND PERIPHERAL NERVOUS SYSTEMS

The nervous system integrates communication and unification throughout the body. Composed of the brain, spinal cord, and a network of nerves, the nervous system is the most complex organ system in the body.

Organized into two main subdivisions, the nervous system consists of the central nervous system (CNS), composed of the brain and spinal cord, and the peripheral nervous system (PNS), composed of the autonomic system and the somatic system. Their interconnecting functions are instrumental in maintaining homeostasis throughout the body.

AUTONOMIC NERVOUS SYSTEM

The autonomic nervous system (ANS) functions at the reflex and subconscious level. It controls the activities of effector organs (muscle, vessel, and gland cells), and its major task is to regulate heart beat, respiration, perspiration, smooth muscle, cardiac muscle, and glandular secretions.

Two opposing subsystems constitute the ANS: the sympathetic system and the parasympathetic system (Fig. 2.3). The sympathetic system consists of thoracic and lumbar nerves along the spinal cord. By dominating during stressful situations, it is known as the emergency "flight or fight" system. The parasympathetic system consists of cranial nerves 3, 7, 9, and 10, and sacral spinal nerves 2 through 4. Its task is to conserve body functions and resources. It dominates during nonstressful situations. A balance of body equilibrium (homeostasis) is maintained through dual innervation of the sympathetic and parasympathetic systems (Table 2.1).

The autonomic motor (efferent) neurons carry impulses from the CNS (brain stem and spinal cord) to the effector organs via ganglions (a network or group of neurons and synapses). Each nerve pathway is subdivided into

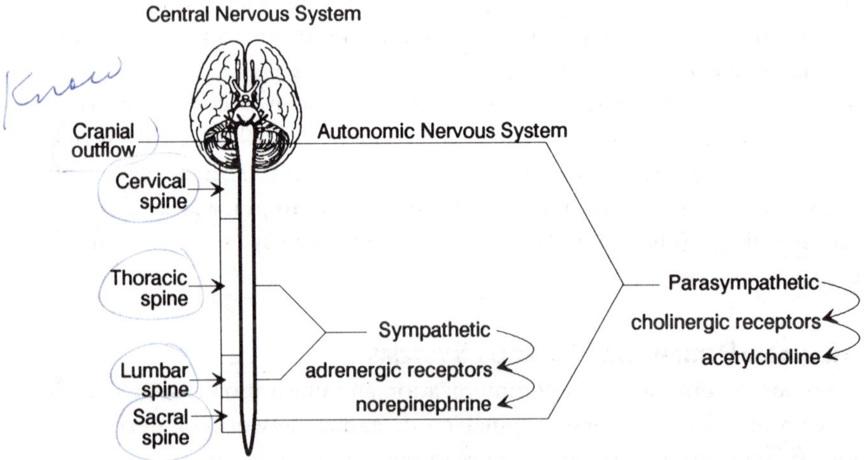

Figure 2.3. Innervation of the sympathetic and parasympathetic systems. See text for explanation.

Table 2.1.
Summary of the Autonomic Functions[a]

Visceral Effector	Adrenergic Response	Cholinergic Response
Heart		
S-A node	Increased rate (β_1)	Decreased rate; vagal arrest
Atria	Increased contractility (β_1)	Decreased contractility
A-V node	Increased conduction (β_1)	Decreased conduction; A-V block
Ventricles	Increased contractility; conduction; automaticity (β_1)	Slight decrease in contractility
Arterioles		
Coronary	Constriction (α) Dilation (β_2)	Dilation
Skin and mucosa	Constriction (α)	Dilation
Skeletal muscle	Constriction (α) Dilation (β_2)	Dilation
Cerebral	Constriction (slight) (α)	Dilation
Pulmonary	Constriction (α) Dilation (β_2)	Dilation
Abdominal viscera	Constriction (α) Dilation (β_2)	—
Salivary glands	Constriction (α)	Dilation
Renal	Dilation (β_1, β_2) Constriction (α)	—
Veins (Systemic)	Constriction (α) Dilation (β_2)	—
Lung		
Tracheal and bronchial muscle	Relaxation (β_2)	Contraction
Bronchial glands	Decreased secretion (α) Increased secretion (β_2)	Stimulation
Salivary glands	Potassium and water secretion (α) Amylase secretion (β)	Potassium and water secretion (strong effect)
Lacrimal glands	—	Secretion
Nasopharyngeal glands	—	Secretion

[a]Slightly modified from Weiner N, Taylor P. Neurohumoral Transmission. In Gilman AG, Goodman LS, Rall TW, Murad F. *Goodman and Gilman's The Pharmacological Basis of Therapeutics.* 7th ed, New York: Macmillan, 1985. Used with permission.

Table 2.1.—*Continued*

Visceral Effector	Adrenergic Response	Cholinergic Response
Pineal gland	Melatonin synthesis (β)	—
Posterior pituitary	Antidiuretic hormone secretion (β_1)	—
Fat cells	Lipolysis (α, β_1)	—
Pancreas		
Acini	Decreased secretion (α)	Secretion
Islets	Decreased secretion (α)	—
	Increased secretion (β_2)	—
Liver	Glycogenolysis and gluconeogenesis (α, β_2)	Glycogen synthesis
Skeletal muscle	Increased contractility; glycogenolysis; potassium uptake (β_2)	—
Adrenal medulla	—	Secretion of epinephrine and norepinephrine
Spleen capsule	Contraction (α)	—
	Relaxation (β_2)	
Skin		
Pilomotor muscles	Contraction (α)	—
Sweat glands	Localized secretion (α)	Generalized secretion
Sex organs (male)	Ejaculation (α)	Erection
Uterus	Pregnant: contraction (α)	Variable
	Relaxation (β_2)	
	Nonpregnant: relaxation (β_2)	
Ureter		
Motility and tone	Increase (α)	Increase (?)
Urinary bladder		
Detrusor	Relaxation (β)	Contraction
Trigone and sphincter	Contraction (α)	Relaxation
Kidney	Renin secretion (β_1)	—
Gall bladder and ducts	Relaxation (β_2)	Contraction
Intestine		
Motility and tone	Decrease (α, β_1, β_2)	Increase
Sphincters	Contraction (α)	Relaxation
Secretion	Inhibition (?)	Stimulation

Table 2.1.—*Continued*

Visceral Effector	Adrenergic Response	Cholinergic Response
Stomach		
Motility and tone	Decrease (α, β_2)	Increase
Sphincters	Contraction (α)	Relaxation
Secretion	Inhibition (?)	Stimulation
Eye		
Radial muscle (iris)	Contraction (α)	—
Sphincter muscle (iris)	—	Contraction
Ciliary muscle	Relaxation (β)	Contraction

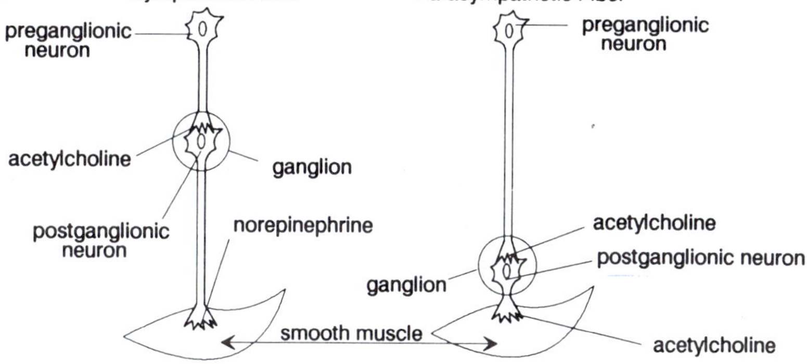

Figure 2.4. The sympathetic and parasympathetic fibers innervating smooth muscle.

preganglionic, ganglionic, and postganglionic neurons (Fig. 2.4). Preganglionic neurons transmit impulses from the CNS to the ganglion. Postganglionic neurons transmit impulses from the ganglion to the effector organ.

Two primary neurotransmitter substances have been documented that conduct impulses at the synapses of the ANS: acetylcholine and norepinephrine. Both the sympathetic and parasympathetic systems contain acetylcholine at all ganglionic synapses. In the parasympathetic system, postganglionic fibers store and ultimately release acetylcholine. In the sympathetic system, the neurotransmitter norepinephrine is stored in the postganglionic fibers (an exception is the postganglionic fibers that innervate the sweat glands and blood vessels of skeletal muscles, in which acetylcholine is the neurotransmitter).

These specific neurotransmitters of the ANS are of major importance and account for the different effects exerted on the effector organs by the sympathetic and parasympathetic systems.

Read Various studies indicate that there may be a third efferent fiber that stores and releases a substance referred to as vasoactive intestinal peptide (VIP) (Hökfelt et al, 1980; Iversen, 1984). It is believed that this peptide either acts as a neurotransmitter or modulates neurotransmission. VIP has the ability to stimulate and activate the adenylate cyclase system, which accounts for most of its activities. Besides being a potent vasodilator, VIP enhances cardiac contractility, stimulates glycogenolysis, and relaxes smooth muscle of the gastrointestinal tract. VIP nerve fibers found in the tracheobronchial tree may control vascular and smooth muscle tone within the airways, inducing vasodilation and bronchodilation. Owing to its ability to induce bronchodilation, VIP may be the forerunner of future types of bronchodilators (pending further investigation).

Synthesis of the Neurotransmitters

There are several natural processes that occur within the postganglionic fiber before norepinephrine and acetylcholine are evolved and thereby taken into their specific storage sites in the postganglionic fiber.

The first step in the synthesis of norepinephrine involves phenylalanine, which is converted to tyrosine by a hydroxylase enzyme. Tyrosine is transported into the cytoplasm of the axon, where it is converted by cytoplasmic enzymes to dopa and then to dopamine. Dopamine is then transported into small sacs (storage vesicles), where the synthesis and ultimate storage of norepinephrine takes place. Norepinephrine is the immediate precursor of epinephrine.

Of interest is the fact that all three of the natural catecholamines (sympathomimetic amines that mimic sympathetic action)—epinephrine, norepinephrine, and dopamine—are involved, at one time or another, in the transmission of sympathetic impulses. Epinephrine is the major hormone of the adrenal medulla, whereas norepinephrine is the primary transmitter of the sympathetic postganglionic fiber. Dopamine is predominantly located in the basal ganglia of the CNS. Dopaminergic fibers and specific receptors for this catecholamine have also been identified in postsynaptic effectors of renal and mesenteric vessels.

The enzyme that initiates the synthesis of acetylcholine in the postganglionic fiber is choline acetyltransferase. Choline acetyltransferase is produced within the cell body of the neuron, then transported to the terminal portion of the axon. Already located in the terminal portion of the axon are a large number of mitochondria, in which the synthesis of acetyl coenzyme A (CoA) takes place. When choline is brought into the cytoplasm (by active transport) from the extracellular fluid, choline acetyltransferase catalyzes the acetylation of choline with acetyl CoA. This final merging of enzymes takes place within the cytoplasm, following which acetylcholine is taken into the storage vesicles.

Figure 2.5 presents a graphic summary of the synthesis of norepinephrine and acetylcholine.

The Autonomic Receptor Theory

The autonomic receptor theory states that when a neurotransmitter substance is liberated from a nerve ending, crosses the synaptic cleft and attaches to a receptor site, a reaction in the target cells is produced.

Receptors that respond to norepinephrine, epinephrine, or similar agents are termed adrenergic. There are adrenergic receptors located on leukocytes, tissue cells, bronchial mast cells, and bronchial smooth muscle. Adrenergic receptors are the primary receptors located throughout the sympathetic system.

Likewise, all receptors that respond to acetylcholine are termed cholinergic. There are cholinergic receptors located at the ganglionic synapses of both the sympathetic and parasympathetic systems. Acetylcholine is also the neurotransmitter of postganglionic fibers that innervate the sweat glands and blood

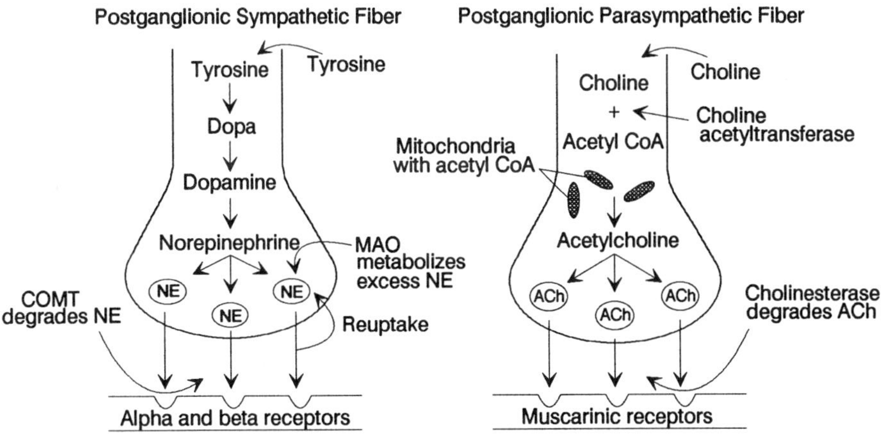

Figure 2.5. The synthesis, storage, release, and inactivation of norepinephrine (*NE*) and acetylcholine (*ACh*). *COMT*, catechol-O-methyltransferase.

vessels of skeletal muscles in the sympathetic system. Cholinergic receptors are located at the neuromuscular junction of skeletal muscle and, finally, cholinergic receptors are the primary receptors located throughout the parasympathetic system.

The Sympathetic System

In the sympathetic system, adrenergic receptors are of two primary types: α and β. There are two subtypes of the α-adrenergic receptor: α_1 and α_2. α_1 Receptors are primarily located at postsynaptic effector sites of smooth muscle and gland cells, whereas α_2 receptors are located on presynaptic nerve terminals. α_2 Receptors are also present at postsynaptic sites in several tissues (e.g., the brain, uterus, and parotid gland) and various regions of vascular smooth muscle.

β Receptors are also subdivided into two types: β_1 and β_2. β_1 Receptors are predominantly located in postsynaptic effector cells of cardiac tissues, while β_2 receptors are present mainly in the postsynaptic effectors of smooth muscle and gland cells.

The activation of α receptors by a neurotransmitter or by α-adrenergic agonists generally induces excitation in the effector site (e.g., mucosal constriction, bronchoconstriction, peripheral vasoconstriction). An exception to this is noted in the intestine, where activation of the α receptors causes relaxation.

Stimulation of β_1 receptors by a neurotransmitter or by β_1-adrenergic agonists results in lipolysis and cardiostimulation (increase in heart beat and contractility). Stimulation of β_2 receptors by a neurotransmitter or by β_2-adrenergic agonists (see also Chapter 8) results in relaxation of smooth muscle tissue (vasodilation and bronchodilation).

This is why the sympathetic system, in particular the β_2-adrenergic receptor site, is the source for respiratory pharmacological manipulation. Fig. 2.6 presents a summary of the pharmacological effects of adrenergic agonists.

Antiadrenergic Drugs that bind to adrenergic receptors and thereby inhibits a neurotransmitter's action on these receptors induce an adrenergic blockade at that site. For example, propranolol (Inderal) is the prototype β blocker used in the treatment of irregular heart beat and hypertension. Inderal is a nonselective β blocker that causes both β_1 and β_2 blockade. (see also Antiadrenergic Action for further discussion of adrenergic blockade.)

As noted previously, different medians act to terminate the action of a neurotransmitter at a receptor site. Liberated norepinephrine in the synaptic cleft is degraded by the enzyme catechol-O-methyltransferase (COMT). COMT has the ability to destroy all catecholamines; therefore, their duration

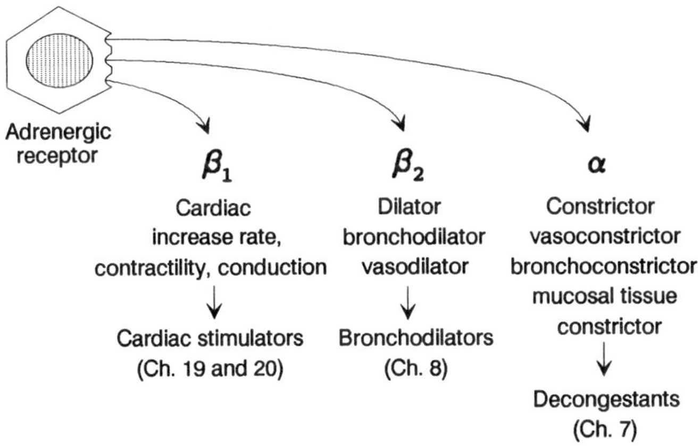

Figure 2.6. Primary effects of adrenergic agonists.

of action is short. Also, if reuptake of norepinephrine into the presynaptic neuron occurs, it is rapidly degraded by the enzyme monoamine oxidase (MAO) (see also Fig. 2.5). When these events occur, the impulse is aborted and the neuron returns to its resting state.

The Parasympathetic System

In the parasympathetic system, cholinergic receptor response to acetylcholine stimulation is similar to the effects produced by muscarine (an alkaloid obtained from various mushrooms, e.g., *Amanita muscaria*). Muscarine exerts its influence only on the smooth muscles, cardiac muscles, and exocrine glands innervated by the parasympathetic system. For this reason, the effects of acetylcholine on the parasympathetic effector cell are designated as muscarinic effects. This term is used in describing the effects of acetylcholine in the parasympathetic system because muscarinic actions on nerve transmission was studied long before acetylcholine was identified. The parasympathetic cholinergic receptor response to acetylcholine is summarized in Table 2.2.

The effects of acetylcholine on cholinergic receptors other than those located at the parasympathetic neuroeffector site (e.g., the autonomic ganglionic synapses, the adrenal medulla, the neuromuscular synapses) are similar to the effects produced by the drug nicotine. Therefore, the effects of acetylcholine on the cholinergic receptors located outside the parasympathetic system and those located at the autonomic ganglionic synapses are designated as nicotinic effects. Along with muscarinic effects, nicotinic effects of acetylcholine are summarized in Table 2.2.

Table 2.2.
Muscarinic and Nicotinic Actions of Acetylcholine

Visceral Effector	Muscarinic Effects	Nicotinic Effects
Cardiovascular blood vessels	Dilation	Constriction
Heart rate	Decrease (via vagus nerve—X cranial)	Increase
Blood pressure	Decrease	Increase
Bronchioles	Constriction	—
Bronchial gland secretion	Increase	—
Gastrointestinal tone	Increase	Increase
Motility	Increase	Increase
Sphincters	Relaxed	—
Glandular secretion	Increase	Initially increase, then decrease
Skeletal muscle	—	Contract
Autonomic ganglia	—	Stimulate
Competitive inhibitor	Atropine	Tubocurarine Pancuronium

The action of acetylcholine at the cholinergic receptor site is terminated through hydrolysis by the enzyme acetylcholinesterase. The duration of action of acetylcholine at nicotinic receptor sites may be prolonged by drugs that have the ability to block the actions of acetylcholinesterase (see Chapter 10).

Competitive inhibition is a term that describes a drug (antagonist) that combines with and occupies a receptor site, thereby preventing an agonist from stimulating this receptor. Atropine (see Chapter 9) is such an antagonist and exerts its opposing effect on muscarinic receptors (see Fig. 9.1). Tubocurarine and pancuronium (see Chapter 11) are examples of nicotinic antagonists (see Fig. 11.3).

MECHANISM OF ACTION WITHIN THE AUTONOMIC NERVOUS SYSTEM

Drug action is the event that occurs when a drug combines with a specific receptor. Drug effect inherently follows drug action. Depending on the number of receptors stimulated, drug effect may be local, systemic, or both. The goal of respiratory drugs is to produce a local effect (lungs) with a twofold approach: to relieve bronchoconstriction and to aid in the clearance of excess secretions by stimulating mucociliary transport.

Normal bronchomotor tone is maintained through the equal opposing forces of the sympathetic and parasympathetic systems. In respiratory disease states the balance of tone is weakened, allowing one system to override the other. β-Adrenergic and anticholinergic drug intervention attempts to return equilibrium to bronchial tone through stimulation of the β-adrenergic receptor or by inhibiting the cholinergic receptor. This is the basis for respiratory pharmacology, and all sympathomimetic and parasympatholytic drug interactions occur at this fundamental level.

Adrenergic Action (Sympathomimetic)

A drug or neurotransmitter that stimulates a β-adrenergic receptor binds to and activates the intracellular enzyme adenylate cyclase. Activated adenylate cyclase catalyzes the conversion of adenosine triphosphate (ATP) to cyclic 3′,5′-adenosine monophosphate (cAMP). The intracellular level of cAMP is important in enhancing the effect of the drug that is bound to the receptor. Bronchomotor tone is influenced by cAMP activating a variety of other intracellular enzyme systems (kinases). The primary effect produced on smooth muscle cells is relaxation (bronchodilation). cAMP also initiates a series of events in the mast cells that lead to inhibition of the release of histamine (a bronchoconstrictor) by suppressing mast cell degranulation.

Stimulation of α receptors opposes the production of cAMP. By inhibiting the adenylate cyclase system, α receptors mediate bronchoconstriction and vasoconstriction.

cAMP is metabolized by the intracellular enzyme phosphodiesterase into the inactive nucleotide 5′-adenosine monophosphate (5′-AMP). If follows then that drugs that prevent the degradation of cAMP by competitively inhibiting phosphodiesterase will prolong the effect and concentration of cAMP. For many years the methylxanthines were thought to be potent phosphodiesterase inhibitors. However, recent studies indicate that theophylline may exert its bronchodilating effect through a different mechanism of action (see Chapter 12).

As noted previously, norepinephrine (a catecholamine by its structure containing a benzene ring, two hydroxyl groups, and an amine side chain) is deactivated by the enzymes COMT and MAO. All catecholamines are deactivated by COMT and MAO. Therefore, the action of any catecholamine is of short duration. Since the concentration of cAMP has a direct cause-and-effect relationship to a bound drug at the receptor site, when the stimulation of a β_2-specific catecholamine is terminated, so also is the production of cAMP.

β_2-Specific drugs that are not catecholamines and therefore are not metabolized by COMT and MAO are of special interest because of their longer duration of action at the β receptor site. Such drugs include the resorcinol and saligenin groups of bronchodilators (see Chapter 8).

Adrenergic drugs work in one of two ways. Either the drug stimulates the release of the natural neurotransmitter norepinephrine from its storage site in the postganglionic fiber (indirectly acting sympathomimetic) or the drug itself exerts its influence on the β receptor site by mimicking the action of the natural neurotransmitter (direct acting sympathomimetic). Primarily, bronchodilators (direct and indirect) either cause an increase in the concentration of cAMP or inhibit the deactivation of cAMP. The result is the same from each action: bronchodilation and vasodilation.

Antiadrenergic Action (Sympatholytic)

Adrenergic blocking agents interfere with the action of norepinephrine, epinephrine, and other sympathomimetics by occupying the α and β receptor sites. Stimulation to or binding of these sites by any sympathomimetic is prevented.

α-Blocking agents are used mainly to increase peripheral blood circulation and to decrease blood pressure. (Remember, α stimulation causes increased peripheral vascular resistance—constriction of blood vessels—and hypertension. Inhibition of α receptors to norepinephrine and sympathomimetics will naturally cause the opposite effect.) Phenoxybenzamine (Dibenzyline) is an α blocking agent used to increase blood flow to the skin and mucosa of patients with peripheral vascular disease and those exposed to frostbite. Phentolamine (Regitine Mesylate) is another α blocking agent that shows promising use for chronic asthma. It produces vasodilation, along with a mild influence on β_2 receptors. IV Mesylate has also been used to treat sympathomimetic drug abuse in which an MAO-inhibitor hypertensive crisis exists (still investigational).

β-Blocking agents combine with β receptors to block the stimulation of epinephrine and adrenergic drugs. β_1 Blockade causes a decrease in the heart rate, decreased contractility, and a decreased cardiac output. β_2 Blockade initiates increased airway resistance in bronchi and inhibits the vasodilating effects of epinephrine on the peripheral blood vessels. β Blockers are used to treat hypertension, cardiac arrhythmias, and myocardial infarction. Inderal, as noted previously, is such a β blocker. β Blocking agents may act upon either β_1 or β_2 receptors or both.

Cholinergic Action (Parasympathomimetic)

The counterpart and opposing force to cAMP is cGMP. Normal bronchomotor tone is mediated intracellularly when these opposing systems are in equal balance (Fig. 2.7).

A drug or neurotransmitter (acetylcholine) that stimulates a cholinergic receptor site binds to and activates the enzyme guanylate cyclase. Activated guanylate cyclase catalyzes the conversion of guanosine triphosphate (GTP) to 3′,5′-guanosine monophosphate (cGMP). Structurally, cGMP is similar to cAMP; nevertheless, cGMP produces opposite physiological effects. Active cGMP stimulates smooth muscle cells and mast cells as does cAMP, except cGMP exerts its influence to constrict smooth muscle (bronchoconstriction). In the mast cell, cGMP enhances the release of histamine by allowing mast cell degranulation. Direct cholinergic receptor stimulation increases the production of intracellular cGMP.

As noted, acetylcholine is degraded by the enzyme acetylcholinesterase. Drugs that have the ability to inhibit acetylcholinesterase will prolong the action of acetylcholine at the receptor site, thereby increasing the level of cGMP.

Cholinergic drugs fall into two classes: those that imitate the action of acetylcholine (direct acting parasympathomimetics) and those that increase the concentration and effect of acetylcholine at the receptor site by inhibiting acetylcholinesterase (indirect acting parasympathomimetics). Acetylcholinesterase inhibitors are used in the treatment of myasthenia gravis, either to diagnose its presence or to give maintenance therapy. Tensilon, Prostigmin,

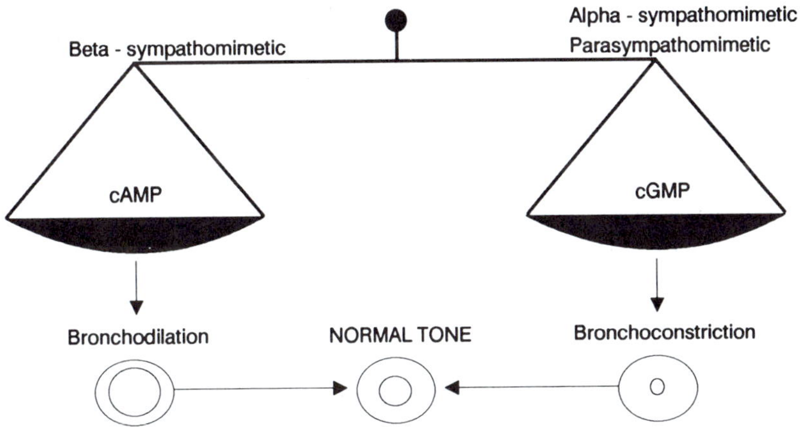

Figure 2.7. Mechanism of bronchial tone.

Mestinon, and Mytelase are indirectly acting cholinergics used in the diagnosis and treatment of myasthenia gravis (see Chapter 10).

cGMP has its own specific phosphodiesterase system, which metabolizes cGMP to its inactive nucleotide 5′-guanosine monophosphate (5′-GMP). Naturally, any drug that acts to stimulate this system will reduce intracellular cGMP, indirectly promoting bronchodilation. Since there are smaller amounts of cGMP than cAMP in muscle cells, the cGMP system is considered less powerful and not as important in respiratory therapeutic manipulation as the cAMP system. The ultimate goal of all bronchodilators (sympathomimetics and parasympatholytics) is to increase intracellular levels of cAMP or to decrease intracellular levels of cGMP, with the primary goal being to enhance the cAMP system.

Anticholinergic Action (Parasympatholytic)

Cholinergic blocking agents prevent acetylcholine from stimulating a cholinergic receptor site through competitive inhibition. Remedial doses of these drugs have little effect on nicotinic sites or at the neuromuscular synapses.

Muscarinic sites of the parasympathetic system are the target receptors for anticholinergics. The primary effect pertaining to the respiratory system that cholinergic blocking agents have is to enhance bronchodilation by reducing the level of intracellular cGMP. The secondary effect is suppression of excessive bronchial mucus secretion. These drugs also depress vagal impulses to the heart, resulting in an increased heart rate. Aerosol inhalation of atropine sulfate is the anticholinergic drug of choice used to relieve cholinergic-mediated bronchospasm and to reduce bronchial secretions (see Chapter 9). An atropine derivative, ipratropium bromide (Atrovent), is available in a metered dose inhaler (MDI) form and is also indicated for relief of bronchospasm. Other uses for atropine include the treatment of hypotensive bradycardia (see Chapter 19) and as a preoperative drying agent for salivary glands.

Figure 2.8 presents a graphic summary of the primary agents and mediators influencing airway activity as they pertain to the cAMP and cGMP systems.

Mediators Influencing Bronchomotor Tone

As mentioned above, normal bronchomotor tone is maintained through the equal opposing forces of the sympathetic and parasympathetic systems. Various types of mediators exist that also play vital roles in airway caliber. Among these are the mast cell mediators, which include those pre-formed within the mast cell itself and those synthesized after mast cell degranulation.

Located throughout the tracheobronchial tree, the mast cell contains many of the mediators of inflammation and bronchoconstriction. The membrane itself contains numerous binding sites for the antibody immunoglobulin E (IgE). When bound to the mast cell, IgE has the unique capability of triggering the release of mediators on contact with antigen, causing an immediate hypersensitivity reaction (see Chapter 13). Various physical and chemical stimuli also trigger the release of mediators from the mast cell (such as exercise, trauma, injury, chemical irritation, and drugs).

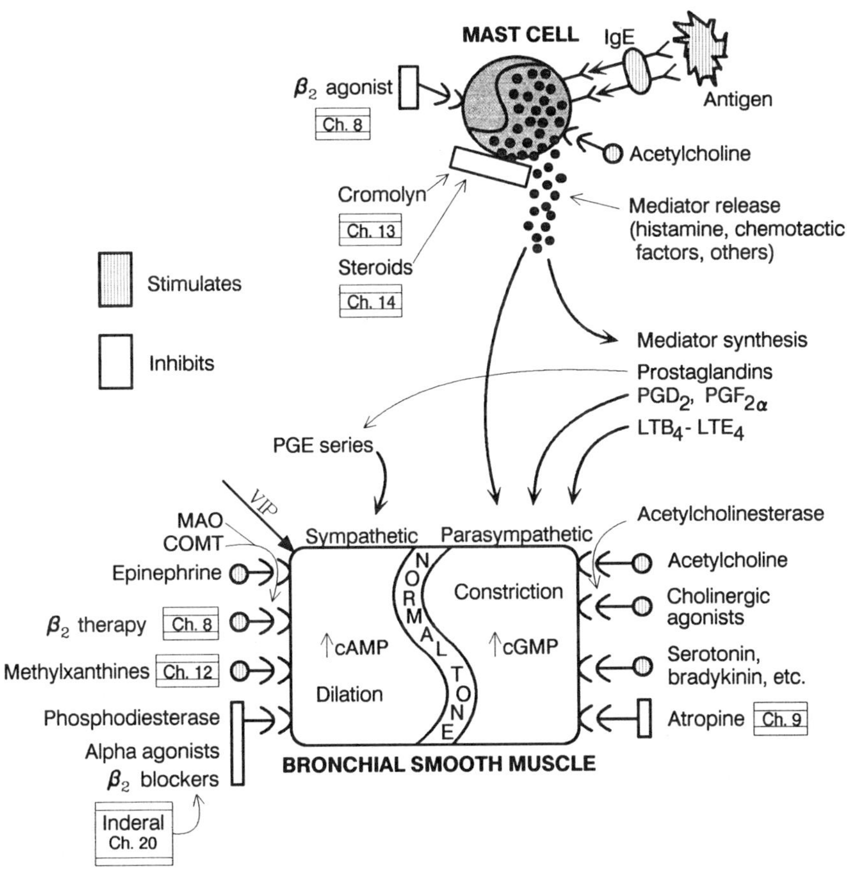

Figure 2.8. Consolidated diagram of airway activity involving endogenous mediators and therapeutic mechanisms of action (with chapter references).

Activation of the mast cell causes the release of histamine. Released histamine acts on and binds to two separate and distinct receptors: $\mathbf{H_1}$ and $\mathbf{H_2}$. Activation of H_1 receptors elicits bronchial and intestinal contraction of smooth muscle, increased capillary permeability, and the formation of edema and wheal (see Antihistamines in Chapter 7), whereas activation of H_2 receptors by histamine mediates gastric acid secretion and cardiac acceleration.

Of utmost concern are the symptoms of anaphylactic shock involved with histamine release. Besides being a major contributor of acute allergic reactions, released histamine also causes cutaneous and laryngeal edema (histamine released from mast cells in the skin and mucosa) and hypotension (histamine release shunts blood from large, low-resistance vessels to mucosal and cutaneous capillary beds). Other autacoids that produce effects similar to those of histamine include serotonin and bradykinin.

Other mediators influencing bronchomotor tone include the prostaglandins, thromboxane, and the leukotrienes. The synthesis of prostaglandins, thromboxane, and leukotrienes is initiated through arachidonic acid metabolism, and the lung is the primary site for the biosynthesis of these substances. No other autacoids show more varied effects than these agents of arachidonic acid metabolism.

Various stimuli—including mast cell degranulation, ischemia, hormones, and drugs—activate the release of arachidonic acid from the cell membrane. Once arachidonic acid is released by the cell membrane, it is oxidized by either cyclooxygenase or lipoxygenase.

The lipoxygenase reaction results in the formation of the highly active leukotrienes (Fig. 2.9). Five primary groups of leukotrienes have been identified: LTA through LTE. LTA_4 is an intermediate in the synthesis of the remaining leukotrienes. The leukotrienes C_4 (LTC_4) and D_4 (LTD_4) are collectively known as the active components of **slow reacting substance of anaphylaxis (SRS-A).** LTE_4 is a less active metabolite of LTD_4.

These leukotrienes of SRS-A exert a prominent bronchoconstrictive effect, enhance the responsiveness of bronchi to histamine (LTD_4), induce contraction of gastrointestinal and vascular smooth muscle (LTC_4 and LTD_4), and constrict coronary arteries and skin vessels (also LTC_4 and LTD_4).

Leukotriene B_4 (LTB_4) is a potent chemotactic agent for neutrophils and eosinophils. The mast cell contains, in granule form, both neutrophil and eosinophil chemotactic factors (NCF and ECF), which are released upon mast cell degranulation (see Fig. 2.8). LTB_4 from eosinophils is a prominent mediator of inflammation and can be released during an anaphylactic reaction.

Arachidonic acid oxidized by the cyclooxygenase mechanism results in the

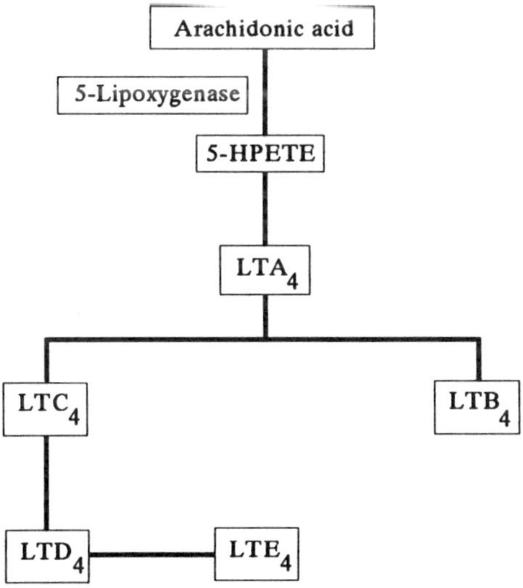

Figure 2.9. Leukotriene synthesis from arachidonic acid.

formation of the prostaglandins and thromboxane (Fig. 2.10). Prostaglandin activity is quite diverse. These agents act on smooth muscle receptors that are not blocked by autonomic blocking agents (such as atropine, propranolol, and phenoxybenzamine). Many actions of the prostaglandins are associated with one of the cyclic nucleotides (cAMP or cGMP).

Prostaglandins $F_{2\alpha}$ ($PGF_{2\alpha}$), D_2 (PGD_2), G_2 (PGG_2), H_2 (PGH_2), and thromboxane (TXA_2) exert bronchoconstrictive effects. $PGF_{2\alpha}$ and PGD_2 are considered the more potent bronchoconstrictors and are of interest as possible mediators of asthma.

Prostaglandins E_1 (PGE_1) and E_2 (PGE_2) stimulate the adenyl cyclase system. The E series of prostaglandins have the ability to relax smooth muscle and suppress the antagonizing effects of bradykinin, histamine, acetylcholine, and serotonin. PGI_2 (prostacyclin) also causes relaxation of bronchiolar smooth muscle.

The bronchodilating prostaglandins may produce new types of bronchodilator agents that will be of interest in the future. However, as it stands, inhaled PGE causes severe irritation of the upper airways or induces paradoxic bronchospasm. Attempts to modify the structure of the PGE series has led to its diminished potency as a bronchodilator. Research and investigation is still being conducted in this therapeutic area. Of interest is the investigation of the analogs of prostacyclin (PGI_2). These agents might be used to prevent the

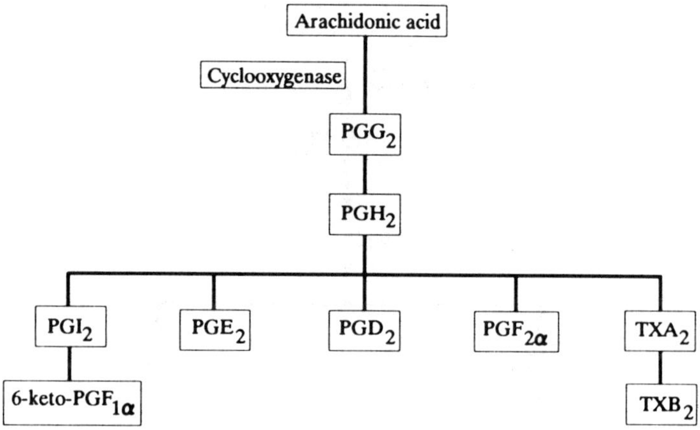

Figure 2.10. Prostaglandin synthesis from arachidonic acid.

bronchoconstricting effects of LTC_4 by inhibiting the conversion of LTA_4 to LTC_4 (a component of SRS-A).

Nonsteroidal antiinflammatory agents (including aspirin and ibuprofen) have the ability to block the synthesis of prostaglandins through the inhibition of arachidonic acid metabolism by the cyclooxygenase pathway. These agents do not affect the lipoxygenase pathway; therefore the leukotrienes are not affected. However, the glucocorticoids (see Chapter 14) have the ability to inhibit the synthesis of both prostaglandins and leukotrienes and are therefore of interest as indirect bronchodilators.

Phases of Drug Events 3

To enhance the comprehension of drug action and effect, a three-phase sequence of events has been developed (Ariens and Simonis, 1974). This chapter focuses on the pharmaceutical phase (drug administration), which deals with the entry route of a drug, and the pharmacokinetic phase, which involves the movement of a drug within the body from the initial absorption by the bloodstream to excretion from the body. (The pharmacodynamic phase, the actual mechanism of drug action and effect within the autonomic nervous system, is presented in Chapter 2.) Figure 3.1 presents an overview of these three phases of drug events. The chapter concludes with a discussion of the nonrespiratory functions of the lungs as they pertain to synthesis, filtration, metabolism, and elimination.

Objectives

1. Identify the primary factors involved when determining the route of drug administration.
2. List the major routes of drug administration. Compare/contrast the intravenous route with the inhalation route.
3. Discuss the advantages and disadvantages of each route of drug administration.
4. State the ideal particle size range for bronchiolar and alveolar deposition. Describe the factors influencing aerosol deposition and the optimal ventilatory pattern to achieve maximal aerosol deposition.
5. Interrelate the various aerosol devices, listing the indication for use and any advantages or disadvantages that may apply.

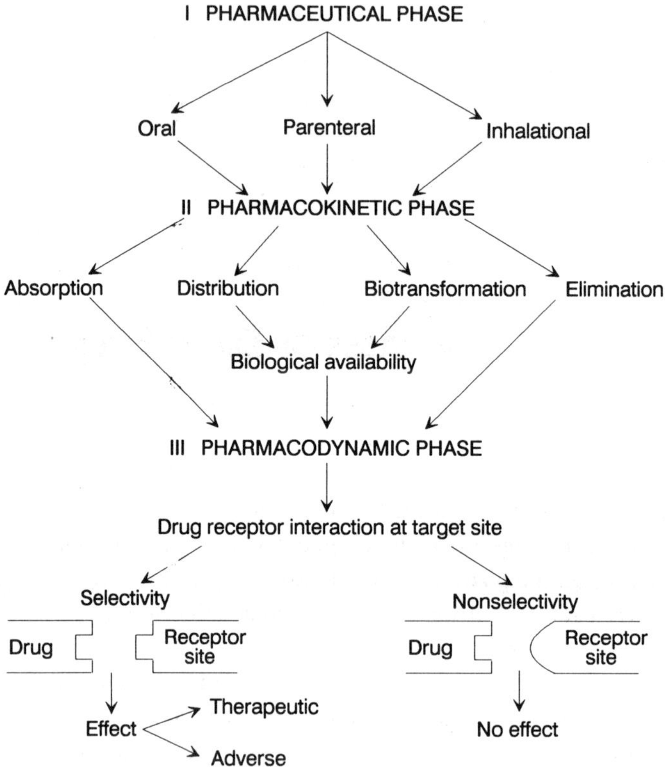

Figure 3.1. The major phases of drug administration, action, and effect, given in sequence.

6. Discuss the process of drug absorption and the factors that influence drug absorption rate. List the four drug transport mechanisms and give a brief explanation of each.
7. Explain the process of drug distribution and redistribution.
8. List the primary organ for drug biotransformation. Also, describe how a drug may be biotransformed and the process that occurs once a drug is biotransformed.
9. Identify the major organ for drug elimination and the factors influencing drug elimination.
10. Describe the various aspects of the lung's nonrespiratory functions as they pertain to synthesis, filtration, metabolism, and elimination.

PHARMACEUTICAL PHASE (DRUG ADMINISTRATION)

Naturally, for a drug to be accessible to the body it must have a route of entry. The dosage form of a drug usually determines the method of administration. For example, pills, tablets, and capsules are inherent to the oral route. When a drug's action and effect are needed immediately, the intravenous route is used. Figure 3.2 compares the various routes of administration.

Other factors to consider pertaining to a drug's route of administration include the extent to which the drug is absorbed and whether either a systemic or a local effect is desired. A patient's age and physical condition also influence the decision of route of drug administration. An unconscious or debilitated patient or a patient who cannot swallow would not be given a tablet or capsule; likewise, an intravenous injection would not be given if another form of drug administration would be more practical, either for economic or emotional reasons. The main and final concern in all routes of administering a drug is the safety of the patient.

Topical Administration

There are two types of topical administration: through the mucous membranes and through the skin.

Topical administration of drugs that are absorbed by the mucous membranes include ophthalmic, nasal, and otic solutions; sublingual and buccal tablets; suppositories; and lozenges. Absorption of drugs through the mucosa occurs

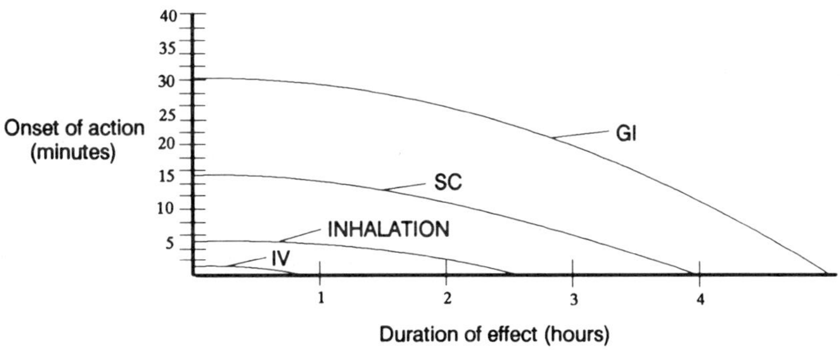

Figure 3.2. Comparison of equal doses of a drug administered by different routes. The intravenous (IV) route achieves the fastest onset of action, followed closely by the inhalation route. The gastrointestinal (GI) and subcutaneous (SC) routes have the slowest onset of drug action; however, drug levels are maintained for a longer period of time.

by diffusion, infiltration, and osmosis. The advantages of mucous membrane absorption include the following:

- Provides quick drug effect—since the mucous membranes are the thinnest, most vascular dermal surface, the drug is absorbed directly into the bloodstream.
- Prevents GI tract irritation.
- May be used if the patient cannot swallow, or if he or she is intubated.
- Avoids degradation by the liver.

The primary disadvantage to topical mucous membrane application is that it may irritate the mucosa.

Topical administration of drugs through skin absorption include lotions, ointments, liniments, powders, and creams. These types of drugs are usually given for their local effect at the site of application. However, if the drug is given for its systemic effect (for example, nitroglycerin transdermal skin patches) the absorption rate is determined by the thickness of the skin layer and by the density of the drug. Advantages of this form of drug administration include:

- Ease of administration;
- Quick relief for itching and pain;
- Fewer allergic or adverse reactions compared to systemic routes.

The primary disadvantage of skin application is adverse reactions to the drug if it becomes systemically absorbed when only a local effect was desired.

Oral Administration

Oral ingestion of drugs is the most ancient method known and still the most commonly used method today. Although the onset of drug action is slow (see Fig. 3.2), oral ingestion is considered to be the safest and most convenient method of drug administration. Oral drug types include capsules, tablets, syrups, elixirs, suspensions (a drug suspended in water), and reconstituted powders and tablets. Advantages to oral administration of drugs include:

- Simplicity and convenience—Most often, the patient may administer the drug himself or herself.
- Safety—Gastric lavage is available in the event of overdosage.
- Economy.

The major disadvantages to oral administration are:

- Slow absorption rate—This factor makes the oral route unsuitable for emergent situations.
- Erratic and incomplete absorption of the drug—Tablets and pills may pass through the GI tract and be excreted in feces undissolved, or form with food substance in the stomach.
- Irritation of the GI tract, emesis—Some forms of liquids and tablets irritate the esophageal mucosa or GI tract, causing emesis. Others may discolor teeth or have an unpleasant taste.
- Possible aspiration—If the patient is debilitated or extremely combative, he or she may accidentally aspirate the drug.
- Drug abusers—Patients with a history of drug abuse may not be able to manage their own therapy and control intake.

Parenteral Administration

Parenteral administration pertains to all injectable drugs given by any route other than through the alimentary canal. Several parenteral forms of drug administration exist; however, the three most commonly used parenteral routes indicated for cardiopulmonary drug administration are presented here (Fig. 3.3).

Intravenous Injection

Intravenous (IV) injection is the most reliable and fastest method of administering drugs directly into the bloodstream. Absorption factors are circumvented, allowing accurate control and titration of drugs. Medications given intravenously should be considered as the route of choice:

- To immediately treat life-threatening conditions and in all emergent situations.

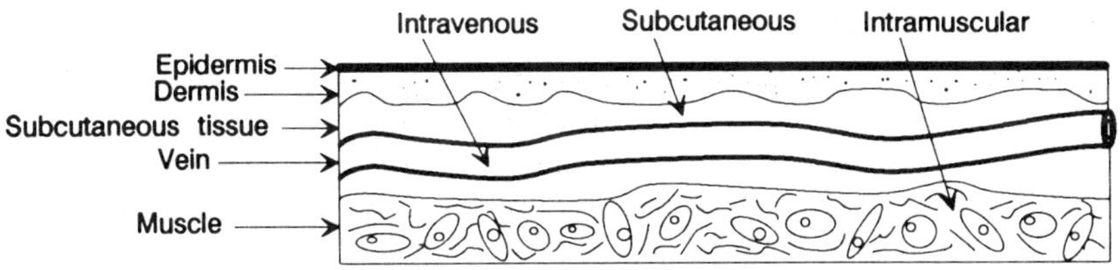

Figure 3.3. The three major injection routes.

- To deliver medications that cannot be given by any other route (e.g., dopamine hydrochloride).
- To delay drug deactivation by the liver.
- To deliver large doses of medication.
- To treat patients who cannot receive medications by any other route (one who is unconscious, patients with gastric ulcers).

There are three methods of IV administration:

Direct administration (IV bolus)—delivers a drug rapidly. The drug becomes effective immediately.

Continuous drip administration (primary line infusion)—maintains drug delivery at a therapeutic level.

Intermittent administration (additive set infusion)—allows the dosage of a drug to be intermittently infused over a period of time, or given as a one time dose.

IV drug administration has several advantages:

- Immediate bioavailability—the drug is injected directly into the bloodstream.
- Dosage is complete and accurate.
- Large drug doses can be delivered.
- Metabolism of the drug by the liver is avoided.

The primary disadvantage of IV drug administration is increased adverse reactions owing to the total direct systemic effect. IV drug administration may cause life-threatening reactions if the drug is delivered too rapidly, if the flow rate is not carefully monitored, or if incompatible drugs are mixed together. Complications such as air embolism, systemic infection, or vein irritation may also occur.

Intramuscular Injection

Intramuscular (IM) injection produces a slower onset of drug action than does the intravenous route; however, drug levels are preserved for longer periods of time. If the general circulation is patent, effective dosages are more predictable. Medications administered through the IM route are usually aqueous suspensions, solutions in oil, or medications that are not available in oral form. An advantage of the IM route over other parenteral routes is that muscles have a greater supply of blood vessels and fewer sensory nerve endings. Other advantages of using the IM route include:

- Allows long-term absorption of medications.
- Allows large doses to be administered (up to 5 ml).
- Does not require an IV injection site.
- Allows medication delivery to a patient who is unconscious, uncooperative, or unable to swallow.

Disadvantages include:

- Slow absorption rate if the medication precipitates in the muscle or if there is a poor blood supply to the muscle.
- Local pain and tissue irritation.
- Possible injection into a nerve, vein, or bone.

Subcutaneous Injection

Subcutaneous (SC) injection produces the slowest onset of drug action found in the parenteral system, yet this enhances a sustained effect of the drug's level. Only drugs that do not irritate tissue are used subcutaneously. Most subcutaneously delivered medications are isotonic, nonviscous, and soluble. The primary advantage of the SC route is easy self-administration (e.g., insulin injection). The two primary factors that affect the absorption rate are exercise (increases blood supply to the area, thereby increasing the absorption rate) and injection site trauma (causes the release of histamine, which in turn decreases blood flow and slows the absorption rate).

Inhalation Administration

All bronchodilators may be given by one or more of the routes mentioned above. The inhalation route is preferred because the access to capillary circulation is rapid owing to the large surface area of the pulmonary system, resulting in almost instantaneous absorption of the drug into the bloodstream. Because the drug is inhaled directly into the airway at its desired site of action, adverse reactions are minimal compared to other routes of administration. Since the drug must be delivered to the alveolar membrane to be effective, patients must have reasonable ventilatory capabilities and patent pulmonary capillary blood flow.

There are three primary advantages of giving drugs by the inhalation route:

- The lung's large surface area allows rapid drug absorption and distribution.
- Potent drugs may be given in small doses, minimizing side effects.
- The respiratory route is easily accessible.

There are two primary disadvantages of giving drugs by the inhalation route:

- Patients must cooperate by inspiring deeply, unless they are mechanically ventilated.
- It is impossible to regulate precise dosages owing to the rainout of drug particles. Some drug particles may be deposited in the oropharynx or swallowed.

Several factors must be considered when using inhalational drugs. As mentioned above, the patient must cooperate by inspiring deeply. For an effective treatment, the patient should inspire slowly and deeply through the mouth with a 5- to 10-second inspiratory hold (for maximum drug deposition and distribution throughout the lungs).

The patient's degree of lung congestion is also a major factor when giving inhalational drugs. Naturally, the more congested the lungs, the more difficult it is for the inhaled drug to penetrate the deeper recesses of the lung.

A third factor to consider when giving inhalational drugs is the *size* of the aerosol drug particles, which affects the stability of the particle and drug deposition within the lung. Aerosolized drug particles approximately 10 μm are inhaled and then deposited into the patient's upper airway (pharynx, larynx, trachea), while particles 5 to 2 μm are deposited proximal to alveoli. Drug particles between 2 and 1 μm can enter the alveoli, with 95 to 100% retention of those particles down to 1 μm. Particles 1 to 0.25 μm are generally stable, with minimal settling. Drug particles less than 0.1 μm are inhaled and exhaled without deposition. Figure 3.4 illustrates aerosol deposition according to drug particle size.

Humidity and Aerosol Therapy

Delivering medications by the inhalation route is usually through humidity or aerosol therapy. Several devices are available that aid the practitioner in administering medications to the patient's tracheobronchial tree. A brief review of the primary delivery systems follows.

Humidifiers

Humidity may be termed "invisible moisture"—water in its vaporous or gaseous state. The rationale for humidity therapy is to provide the patient's inspired gases (either oxygen or air) with enough water vapor to make it comfortable to breathe. To increase a humidifier's efficiency, heat is applied, allowing the inspired gases to be fully saturated (100% relative humidity at body temperature). It is essential for every patient whose upper airway is

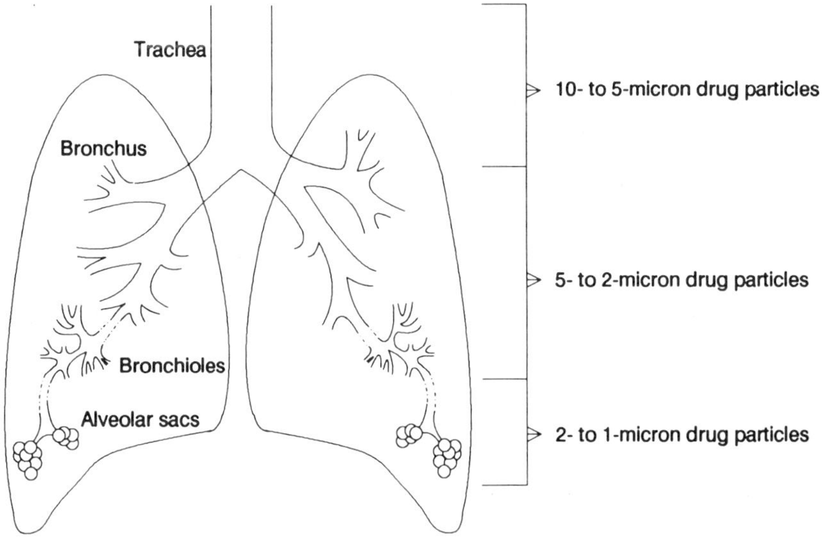

Figure 3.4. Inhaled drug particle deposition. The smaller the drug particle, the better its deposition into the deeper recesses of the lungs.

bypassed—intubated or tracheostomy patients—to have inspired gases at 100% relative humidity at body temperature.

There are several types of humidifiers available for patient use. Probably the most common unit in use is the *bubble humidifier* (also known as a diffuser humidifier). The diffuser head located below the water surface produces small bubbles, thereby increasing the efficiency (humidity output) of the device. The incoming gas flow is directed to the diffuser head, and the resultant humidified gas is then directed to the patient.

Aerosol Devices

The primary method of delivering medications (bronchodilators, mucolytics) by the inhalation route lies with aerosol therapy. An aerosol consists of solid or liquid particles that are suspended in a gas. Inhalation aerosol therapy, therefore, is a suspension of a drug that is dispensed in a spray or mist.

The devices used in aerosol therapy include various types of nebulizers (many are based on the Babington, ultrasonic, Bernoulli, or Venturi principle), which produce aerosol particles for inhalation. A baffle placed within the device reduces the larger particles into smaller ones, thereby allowing deeper deposition into the tracheobronchial tree. If larger particles are desired for deposition into the upper airways an *atomizer* may be used, which is basically a nebulizer without any baffles. Nebulizers are generally powered by a compressed gas source (either oxygen or air). The exception is the ultrasonic nebulizer, which is electrically powered.

Each nebulizer has its own specific indication for use:

- Small volume jet nebulizer (SVN): The SVN is also known as a hand-held nebulizer (HHN) or updraft nebulizer. This device has a reservoir capacity of <20 ml and is indicated for bronchodilator therapy. A disadvantage to the use of this device is medication waste during exhalation. This disadvantage can be eliminated with the use of a finger valve placed in line before the nebulizer. By occluding the orifice during inhalation nebulization is permitted. Releasing the port during exhalation shunts the gas flow to the atmosphere.
- Large-reservoir air-entrainment nebulizer: To provide continuous oxygen therapy with humidity a heated (if 100% body humidity is required) large-reservoir air-entrainment jet nebulizer is used. The reservoir capacity is approximately 250 to 400 ml. Sterile water must be used in this device owing to the particulate water produced (aerosol environments are a source for the colonization and spread of pathogenic bacteria).
- Babington nebulizer (Solosphere, Hydronamic): The Babington nebulizer is indicated as an aid in mobilizing secretions and for sputum induction. To hydrate secretions for expectoration the patient inhales a hypertonic saline solution (or sterile water may be used) for 20 to 30 minutes. Following the treatment, the patient is encouraged to expectorate into a specimen cup. The sputum sample obtained is then sent to the laboratory for analysis.
- Ultrasonic nebulizer (USN): The ultrasonic nebulizer incorporates a piezoelectric transducer that has the ability to change its shape (oscillate) when a current is applied. The aerosol particles produced are in the 1- to 5-μm range, ideally suited for bronchiolar and alveolar deposition. The USN is indicated to facilitate the mobilization of bronchial secretions. This is accomplished by thinning thick, retained secretions. Treatments are usually given for 20 to 30 minutes tid or qid.

Because the Babington and ultrasonic nebulizers deliver highly dense aerosol mists, an inherent hazard to their use is the precipitation of bronchospasm, especially in individuals with hyperreactive airways. An alternative to the use of a hypertonic saline solution or sterile water is normal saline or a hypotonic saline solution, which are less irritating to airways (see also Chapter 15). However, if bronchoconstriction occurs with the use of these nebulizers the treatment must be stopped and safer techniques should be employed.

Metered dose inhalers (MDIs) are pressurized glass, ceramic, or metal canisters containing a drug to be nebulized. A metered-dose aerosol is produced with the use of a propellant and a valve mechanism designed to deliver a specific amount of medication. The propellant is some physiologically inert gas (usually Freon 11 or some other fluorocarbon) that liquefies under pressure.

When the nozzle of the canister is depressed, a fine aerosol spray is released that consists of the drug enclosed within the propellant. As the propellant evaporates the drug remains suspended and continues on in the airstream.

Recent advances in MDI administration include the use of mist-confining (extension devices, holding chambers, spacers) and demand (synchronizes medication discharge with inspiration) systems. Designed to facilitate application and minimize aerosol waste, these devices may provide for a more stable aerosol particle with a deeper penetration into the lungs. These MDI adjuncts are especially beneficial in patients unable to coordinate proper technique.

Dosage is extremely variable depending on patient technique and compliance. Approximately 10 to 20% of all patients do not receive an optimal dose or optimal aerosol deposition due to improper technique. Therefore, it is extremely important for the practitioner to properly instruct the patient on MDI use. Proper technique and application include:

- If using both a bronchodilator and corticosteroid use the bronchodilator first, then the corticosteroid.
- Remove MDI and shake it vigorously. If the device has not been used in over 24 hours, charge the inhaler by holding the canister upside down and actuate by depressing the nozzle.
- Exhale to resting level.
- Open the mouth wide and place the canister, nozzle down, about 1 inch from the mouth, making sure the lips and teeth do not obstruct the aerosol flow. If the lips and teeth are closed around the mouthpiece the aerosol will be deposited mainly in the mouth or hypopharynx.
- Activate the MDI by depressing the nozzle of the canister *after* inspiration has started and maintain a slow deep inspiration.
- Maintain an inspiratory pause of at least 5 to 10 seconds to maximize deposition and distribution of the drug.
- Repeat procedure in 1 to 3 minutes.
- Rinse the mouth and throat with water after use (this is especially important when using corticosteroids due to the risk, although low, of developing an oral fungal infection such as that caused by *Candida albicans.* Use of a spacer

and hyperextending the neck is also recommended to decrease the incidence of fungal infection.)

- Rinse the mouthpiece after each use and disinfect once a week with a solution containing one-half white vinegar and one-half water for approximately 30 minutes, then rinse with water.

MDIs are a popular form of aerosol drug administration owing to their compactness and ease of operation. Commonly prescribed for self-administration and home use, MDIs may be a considerable source for potential abuse among chronic respiratory patients. The practitioner should assume a primary role with these patients in proper education and application.

One final note—Freon propellants have been known to cause life-threatening cardiac arrhythmias. Because of this and due to environmental issues, the use of Freon as a propellant is being reevaluated by manufacturers.

PHARMACOKINETIC PHASE (MOVEMENT OF DRUGS WITHIN THE BODY)

Administering a drug initiates a cycle of physiochemical activities within the body. Absorption, distribution, biotransformation, and elimination are processes involved in the movement of a drug after it is administered to the body (see Fig. 3.5). These factors, plus the route of administration, determine the delivery of a drug to its site of action.

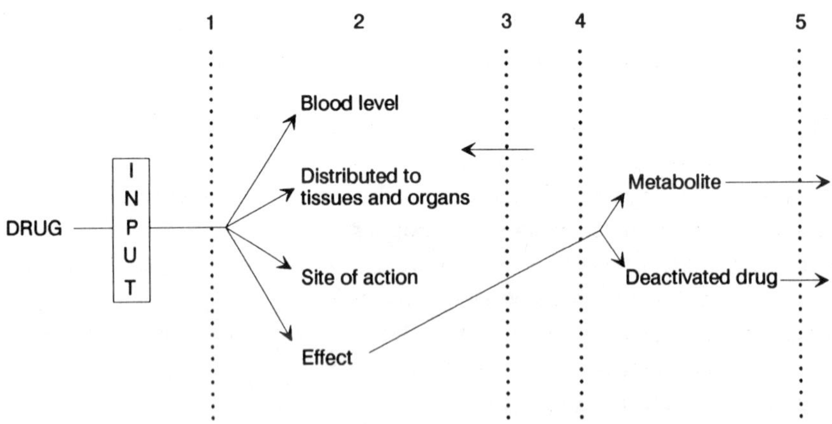

Figure 3.5. 1, Absorption; 2, distribution; 3, redistribution; 4, biotransformation; 5, elimination. See text for explanation.

Absorption

A drug must first be absorbed into the bloodstream before it can gain access to the body's receptor sites. Absorption of a drug and the rate at which this occurs is dependent on several factors. How much of a dose actually gets into the body is the first factor. With intravenous injection, bioavailability of a drug is 100%, owing to the fact that the drug is immediately injected into the bloodstream and bypasses the process of absorption. With other routes of administration, the rate of absorption is dependent on the solubility of a drug (aqueous solutions are absorbed more rapidly than colloids or suspensions) and blood flow within the body. Decreased systemic circulation may slow the rate of absorption, especially if a drug is given subcutaneously. Absorption of inhaled adrenergic drugs occurs through the lung mucosa and the alveolar capillary membrane. Ventilation-perfusion abnormalities and severe diffusion defects of the lung have the greatest effect of slowing the uptake of a drug.

Most of the factors that affect the rate of absorption that have been presented so far are variables that hinder the rate of absorption of a drug. Factors that enhance the rate of absorption are (*a*) increased concentration of a drug, (*b*) increased circulatory blood flow, (*c*) as noted, increased drug solubility, and (*d*) increased area of absorbing surface (such as the pulmonary alveolar epithelium and gastrointestinal tract).

As mentioned, intravenous injection enables a drug to be administered directly into the bloodstream, allowing its absorption to be immediate. However, other drug forms must first penetrate one or more cell-membrane barriers from the administration site to reach the circulatory system. These drugs are allowed to reach the circulatory system by one of four transport mechanisms:

Passive diffusion—The most common transport mechanism. A concentration gradient exists from one side of the cell membrane to the other when a drug is introduced into the body. With no energy expended, the drug diffuses across the cell membrane until the drug concentration equalizes on both sides of the cell membrane.

Facilitated diffusion—Like passive diffusion, facilitated diffusion operates by means of a concentration gradient and also requires no energy expenditure. Drug molecules combine with carrier substances, enabling the drug to penetrate the cell membrane until equal amounts are present on both sides of the cell membrane.

Active transport—This process requires energy because it transfers drug molecules against the concentration gradient. A drug combines with a carrier substance, which takes it from a lower concentrated area to a higher concentrated area.

Pinocytosis—This form of active transport occurs when the cell membrane actually engulfs drug molecules, thereby transporting the drug into the cell. Only a few drug types can be absorbed by this process.

Figure 3.6 presents a graphic representation of these four transport mechanisms.

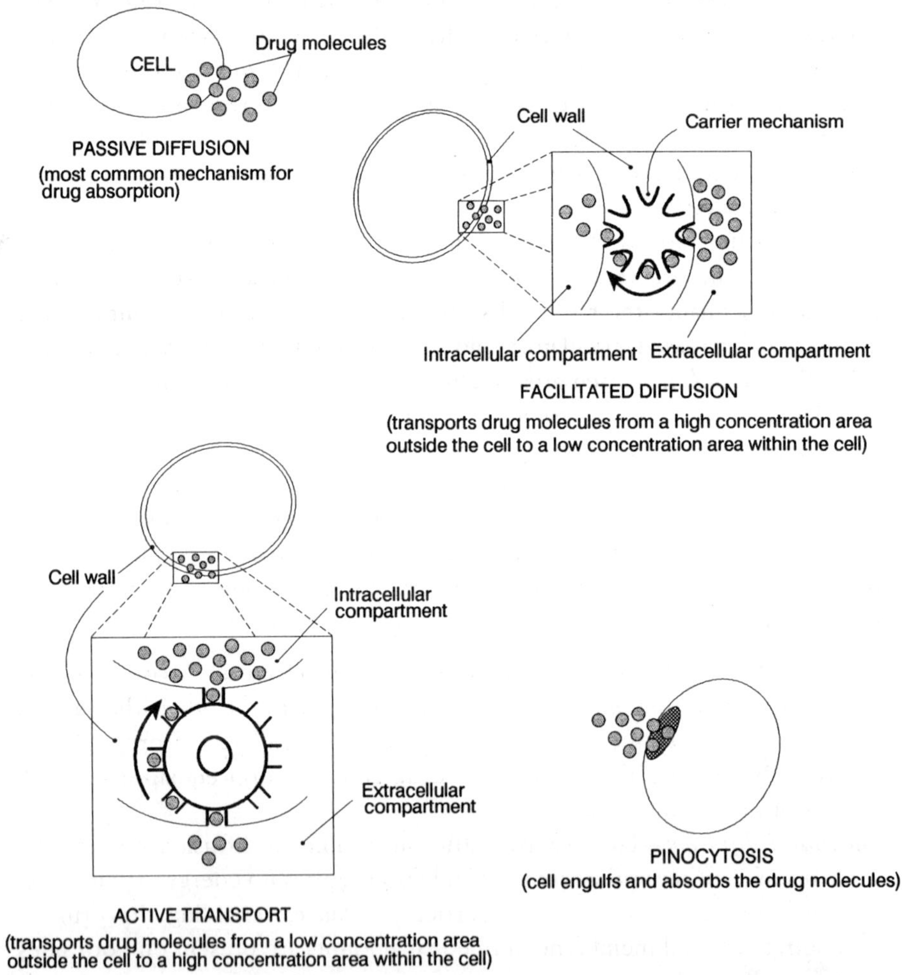

Figure 3.6. Conceptual illustration of the four transport mechanisms. (Adapted from Deglin J, Walters J. *Nursing Now: Drug Interactions*. Springhouse, PA: The Springhouse Corporation, 1984.)

Distribution

Through absorption, a drug is made available to the bloodstream. Through distribution, a drug's site of action is attainable by allowing the drug to traverse the body's circulating bloodstream and be exposed to interstitial and cellular fluids and tissues. The rate and pattern of distribution is determined by the physiochemical effects of the drug, by cardiac output, and by circulatory blood flow.

Of major importance in the distribution of a drug is the systemic and pulmonary blood circulation. How soon a drug reaches its target area depends greatly on blood supply. Highly vascular organs (e.g., heart, liver, kidneys) receive the drug molecules first, whereas it takes longer for the drug to reach less vascular areas (e.g., muscle, fat, skin). It follows then that impairment of perfusion and circulation may lead to the total dose of the drug not being accessible to receptor sites.

As drugs are absorbed into the circulatory system, one of three actions occurs to the drug molecule: drug molecules may become bound to plasma proteins (usually albumin) or red blood cells, or remain free. Both bound and unbound drug molecules traverse the body's circulatory system to reach the fluid compartments and tissues. However, only those drug molecules that remain unbound are able to react with the body's receptor sites and exert a pharmacologic effect.

Plasma protein binding of drug molecules serves as a temporary storage compartment for the drug. As the free drug molecule is metabolized and excreted, the bound drug is gradually released from the plasma protein. This process enables the body to maintain therapeutic drug levels.

When different drug types compete with the same plasma protein, a type of interaction occurs that disturbs the bound/unbound ratio. Either both drugs are not fully bound to the protein or the second drug displaces the first drug. Serious problems occur when a large amount of a bound drug is suddenly displaced from the protein. The patient could well suffer the effects of an overdose.

The extent of protein binding depends on the drug's molecular structure and is a highly variable factor with each drug type. For example, 97% of warfarin sodium (Coumadin, an anticoagulant) binds to plasma proteins when administered to the body. Coadministering a drug such as phenylbutazone (an anti-inflammatory agent) will compete with and displace protein-bound warfarin sodium. Freeing just 3% of warfarin from the protein doubles the amount of active drug within the system, which could easily lead to overdose and possible hemorrhage. Eventually, the body may excrete the excess dose.

Redistribution

The phenomenon of redistribution may occur when a drug is taken back into the bloodstream after stimulating a receptor and is redistributed to other tissues and sites other than the expected site.

Biotransformation

Biotransformation is a word usually interchangeable with metabolism, which basically means any chemical alterations of a compound (e.g., a drug). A metabolite is the by-product of this alteration. Some drugs may continue to be active until they have undergone metabolism. This process enhances the drug's elimination from the body.

Biotransformation of a drug mainly occurs through enzymes located in the liver, but it may also occur in the lungs, kidneys, bloodstream, or intestines. The rate at which biotransformation of a drug occurs is highly variable, depending upon an individual's normal metabolic rate, his age, any genetic disorders, disease, or drugs in his system.

Elimination

A drug may be eliminated from the body chemically unaltered or as a metabolite. The kidneys serve as the most important organ for the excretion of a drug. Excretion of a drug may also occur through perspiration, saliva, tears, or feces. Elimination of a drug by feces is usually unabsorbed orally ingested drugs. Anesthetic gases, paraldehyde, vapors, and aerosols are eliminated through exhalation of the respiratory cycle. Factors hindering drug elimination include interactions with other drugs or impairment of renal, hepatic, or cardiovascular functions.

PHYSIOLOGIC NATURE OF THE LUNGS

Many are aware of the lung's primary function—that of gas exchange. Yet, the lung performs several vital nonrespiratory functions as well.

Synthesis

As mentioned in Chapter 2, the lung is the major site for the synthesis and release of various autacoids. Histamine synthesis occurs in the lung as well as the arachidonic acid metabolites (prostaglandins, thromboxane, leukotrienes).

Certain cells of the lung (e.g., neutrophils and macrophages) complement the synthesis of oxygen-derived free radicals for bactericidal action. Active lung neutrophils and other phagocytes also lead to the release of the proteolytic enzymes elastase and trypsin.

The lung contains a unique transport system to rid itself of these dangerous proteases. These enzymes are transported (via the flow of mucus) to the larynx where the enzymes are conjugated by α_1-antitrypsin. This action forms a detoxified product for elimination through the pulmonary vascular bed and lymph system.

Synthesis of surfactant occurs within the lung by the alveolar (type II) cells. Surfactant has the capacity to reduce alveolar surface tension, enhancing the elasticity of the pulmonary tissue. Liberated surfactant is found throughout the alveoli and respiratory air passages.

Filtration

Because of the unique position of the lung between the venous and arterial circulations, the pulmonary vascular bed has the ability to process and filter various substances, thereby protecting the coronary and cerebral circulations. The large surface area of the pulmonary vascular bed is ideally suited for this task. This filtration process is why there is a difference in blood levels of a substance between venous and arterial samples.

By active uptake, serotonin and epinephrine are removed from the pulmonary circulation, although histamine is relatively unaffected by the lung's filtration process. Many of the prostaglandins, the leukotrienes, and bradykinin are also removed through the pulmonary circulation. PGE, $PGF_{2\alpha}$, and bradykinin are removed during a single pass through the pulmonary circulation, making their duration of action very limited.

Metabolism

Among its various activities, the lungs also have the ability to metabolize various vasoactive substances from blood or tissues. Angiotensin I (a decapeptide hormone) is hydrolyzed by a peptidase located within the lung to angiotensin II, a potent vasopressor and stimulator of aldosterone production and secretion.

The pulmonary system contains an abundant source of thromboplastin and plasmin activator. Thromboplastin aids in the conversion of prothrombin to thrombin, which then coverts fibrinogen to fibrin. Plasmin activator contributes in the dissolution of formed fibrin clots by initiating the conversion of plasminogen to plasmin.

The lung also contains an active cytochrome P-450 enzyme system (a group of hemoproteins), which gives it the ability to biotransform and detoxify many substances, including drugs.

Elimination

Elimination of a substance may occur through the pulmonary circulation as mentioned above or through exhalation of the respiratory cycle. As mentioned earlier, the various inhaled drugs (anesthetic gases, paraldehyde, vapors, and aerosols) are eliminated through exhalation in the respiratory cycle.

Factors that Modify Drug Effects 4

The degree to which a drug produces an effect within the body is dependent on several factors and interacting relationships. Before administering a drug, these factors must be taken into account and the dosage adjusted to meet the specific requirements of individual patients. The more important factors that modify drug effects are represented in Figure 4.1.

Objectives

1. Identify the physiological and pathological variables that modify drug effects.
2. Explain the dose-effect relationship. Interrelate how potency, slope, variability, and maximal efficacy affect the dose-effect relation.
3. Define the terms LD_{50}, TI, ED_{50}, hyperreactive, hyporeactive.
4. Indicate how compensatory reflex affects the autonomic nervous system.
5. Describe biologic half-life, give an example of and the factors affecting biologic half-life of a drug.
6. Define the terms synergism, summation, potentiation.
7. Explain physical antagonism, chemical antagonism, pharmacological antagonism.
8. Define tolerance, tachyphylaxis, cumulation.
9. Specify how age, pregnancy, and allergies affect a drug's dosage.

Physiological Variables

The physical and chemical processes of the body (such as water and electrolyte balance, body temperature, acid-base status, and other physiological variatives)

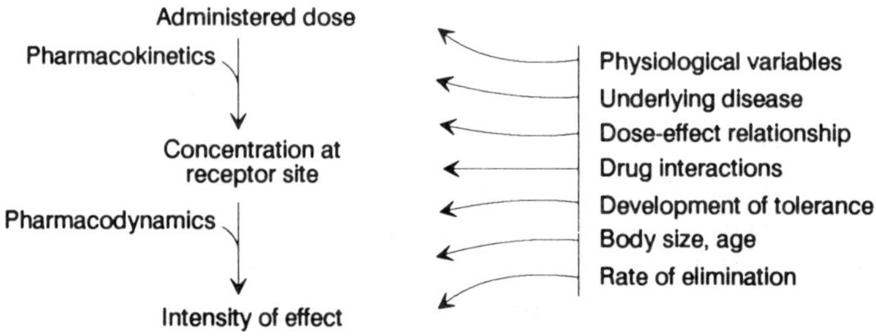

Figure 4.1. Factors that determine the relationship between an administered drug and alterations in expected drug effect.

may alter drug effects. Of special concern to the practitioner is acid-base status. Acidosis, regardless of etiology, may change the protein binding capability of the cell membrane. This limits a portion of the drug available for diffusion out of the capillary and into tissue. This then may lead to a decreased response to adrenergic drugs in the acidemic patient.

PATHOLOGICAL FACTORS

Cardiovascular, renal, hepatic, and pulmonary disease are major pathological factors that modify drug effects. Drug therapy and dosage should be frequently monitored for clinical response and early indications of toxicity.

Renal and hepatic failure alters a drug's absorption, distribution, excretion, and pharmacological response. Since the liver is the major organ for drug biotransformation, it is best to avoid drugs that are metabolized by the liver. Some orally ingested drugs must first pass through the liver before reaching the systemic circulation. IV or IM administration of these drugs should therefore be given priority.

As noted, the kidney is the primary organ for drug excretion. In the presence of renal failure, not only are the metabolic demands of the body not met but there may be an accumulation of administered drugs within the body, creating life-threatening toxic conditions.

Impairment of circulatory blood flow, as with cardiovascular or peripheral vascular disease, has the greatest effect of altering a drug's distribution to its receptor site. In the presence of severe cardiovascular disease a portion of the blood flow is redistributed to vital organs, leaving other organs with inadequate tissue perfusion. With abnormal tissue blood flow, all routes of drug administration may be ineffective other than the intravenous or inhalational routes.

Pulmonary disease has the capability of altering a drug's onset of action and peak effectiveness. Aerosolized drugs are well absorbed by the lung mucosa, and the onset of drug action is rapid if the airway is patent. Lung disease in which there is a large ventilation-perfusion abnormality profoundly affects the absorption of a drug through the alveolocapillary membrane. A quantity of the drug may be lost to the nonperfused, nonventilated areas. Although a quantity of the aerosolized drug may be displaced, it is still an effective means of drug administration, for aerosolized drugs have the advantage of direct utilization to the receptor organ (smooth muscle of the bronchioles).

DOSE-EFFECT RELATIONSHIP

The distribution of a drug throughout the body is not a selective process; however, a drug's ability to stimulate and act upon specific receptor sites is. At reduced dosages a drug may interact with only a few specific receptors, producing a minimum of effects. At higher dosages a drug may interact with more receptors, initiating and intensifying a variety of effects. The relation between the given amount (dose) of a drug and the intensity of the response elicited is referred to as the dose-effect relation (Fig. 4.2). Each effect and the intensity of the response produced at varying dosage levels may be assimilated into a dose-effect curve. Four pertinent components of the curve include *potency, slope, variability,* and *maximal efficacy.*

Potency

Potency is a dose-related occurrence that refers to the amount of a drug required to elicit a certain effect. The lower the dose required to elicit a

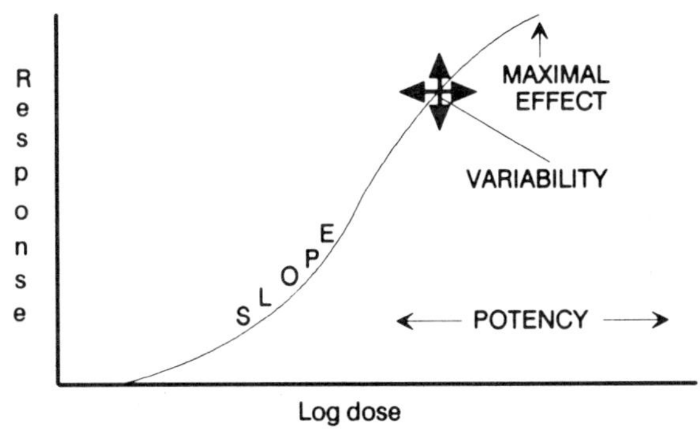

Figure 4.2. The dose-effect relation.

response, the more potent the drug (Fig. 4.3). For a given range of expected responses from a drug, the lowest dose should be administered that will produce the effects desired. Pharmacokinetics, the concentration of the drug, and the drug's intrinsic ability to combine with receptors influence potency. Comparatively, potency (located along the dose axis) does not equate with the degree of effectiveness of a drug; therefore, a highly potent drug may not necessarily be the most effective drug (Fig. 4.4).

Slope

The central, more or less linear portion of the curve forms the slope. A sheer upright slope signifies that maximal effects will be achieved with very small

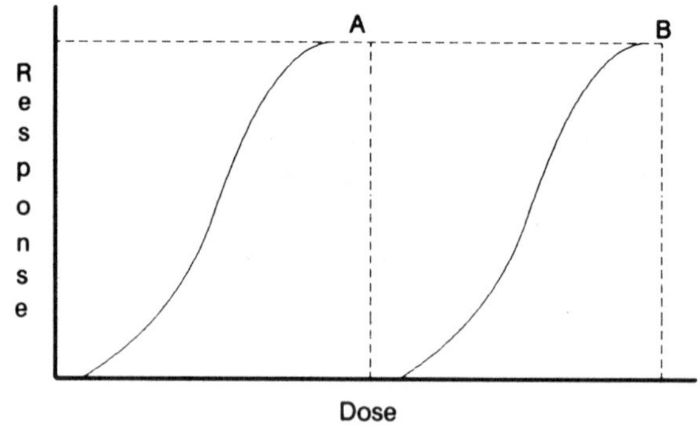

Figure 4.3. Drug A is more potent than drug B because drug A produces its maximal effect at a lower dose.

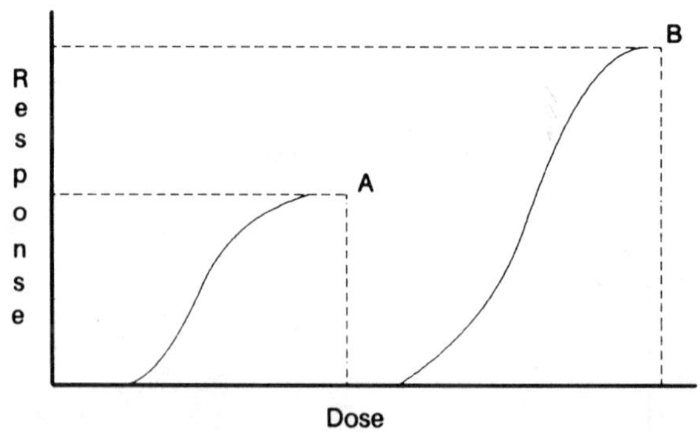

Figure 4.4. Drug A is more potent than drug B because it requires a lower dose to reach maximal efficacy, yet drug B is more effective because it possesses a higher drug efficacy.

increments in dose (Fig. 4.5). It is necessary to be aware of this factor when considering the relative safety of a drug.

Maximal Effect

Intrinsic to a drug is its maximal effect, referred to as drug efficacy. Drugs are inherently capable of generating greater effects; however, as undesired effects limit a drug's dosage, so is its efficacy limited.

Variability

The final component to be considered in the dose-effect relationship is biological variation. Exact drug response is never identical in all patients; therefore a drug's dose produces varying effects in each individual. The median effective dose (ED_{50}) is the dose required to elicit a response in 50% of individuals. Individuals who respond to a lower dosage, compared to the average dose, are said to be hyperreactive. As such, individuals who require a higher than average dose to produce a response to the drug are hyporeactive. Idiosyncrasy refers to an unusual effect generated from a drug that is not related to the dosage or its intensity; this is usually a result of drug allergy. If death is the end effect of a drug, then the median lethal dose (LD_{50}) replaces the median effective dose (Fig. 4.6). Therapeutic index (TI) refers to the relative safety of a drug and is calculated by dividing LD_{50} by ED_{50}. As the index approaches zero, the margin of safety of a drug's given amount of dosage is greatly reduced.

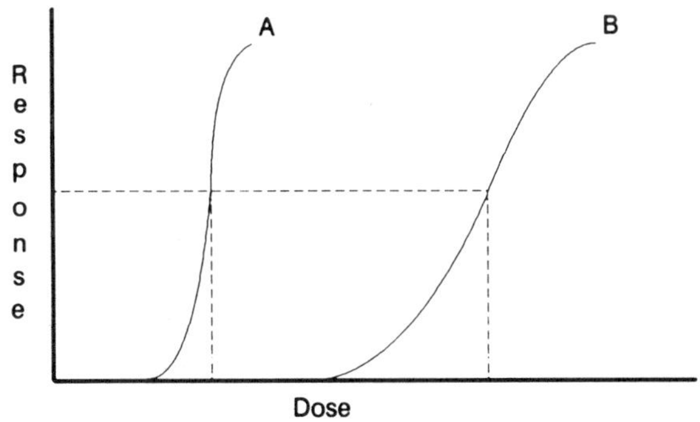

Figure 4.5. Very small increments in dose of drug A (compared to drug B) greatly increases the drug's effect, yet both drugs possess the same maximal efficacy.

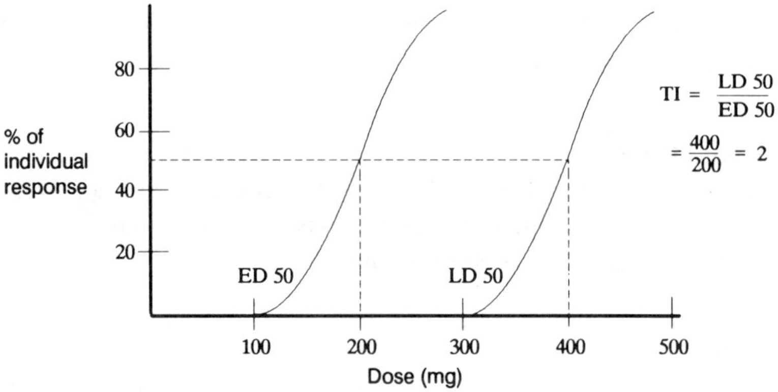

Figure 4.6. For a given increase in the amount of a dose, the median lethal dose (LD_{50}) is observed.

COMPENSATORY REFLEX EFFECTS

Compensatory reflex action of the autonomic nervous system initiates a series of events that lead to a modification in the response to sympathomimetic drugs. Compensatory reflex response determines the sympathetic tone when an α or β receptor site is actuated. For example, the compensatory reflex effect in the cardiovascular system to α-adrenergic stimulation is a rise in blood pressure through constriction of blood vessels. This results in a diminution of sympathetic tone throughout the system that tends to lessen the intensity of the effects produced by sympathomimetic drugs. β-Adrenergic stimulation produces dilation of skeletal muscle blood vessels with corresponding constriction of other vascular beds through compensatory reflex action to maintain equilibrium of the blood pressure. This enhances overall sympathetic tone and the effectiveness of sympathomimetic drugs.

BIOLOGIC HALF-LIFE

Biologic half-life (t½) refers to the time in which 50% of an administered drug is eliminated from the body. Biologic half-life establishes dosage frequency for each particular drug. For example, if it takes 4 hours for a drug to be 50% eliminated from the body, then the drug may be given 6 times per day. Biologic half-life varies with age, body weight, underlying disease, and the presence of other drugs. It is an important factor to be considered in dosing regimens.

DRUG INTERACTIONS

A drug interaction occurs whenever a drug's expected therapeutic effect is restricted, modified, enhanced, or altered in any way by an interactant chemical. The most common interactant is another drug or a combination of drugs (drug-drug interaction). The response to the drug-drug interaction may result in one of three effects: an increase in drug effect, a decrease in drug effect, or an increase in the incidence of an adverse side effect of the drug.

Augmented drug effects caused by an interactant are composed of three types:

Synergism—This occurs whenever the combined effect of two drugs is greater than the sum of their independent effects. For example; coadministered bronchodilators with xanthines produce synergistic activity.

Summation—This occurs whenever the combined effect of two drugs is equal to the sum of their independent effects.

Potentiation—This occurs whenever a drug alters the response of another drug by modifying the initial drug's metabolism, either through absorption, distribution, biotransformation, or excretion. The result usually produced is an additive effect, enhancing the combined drugs' action within the body.

A drug interactant may produce a reduction in drug effect through one or more opposing effects:

Physical antagonism—This occurs whenever a drug physically interacts to reduce the absorption rate of the initial drug.

Chemical antagonism—Two drugs chemically interacting with one another to produce inactive products. This process usually occurs through oxidation or hydrolysis.

Pharmacological antagonism—This occurs whenever two drugs having opposing effects compete for the same receptor site (e.g., the competitive inhibition of atropine and acetylcholine).

OTHER FACTORS THAT MODIFY DRUG EFFECT

Tolerance—This develops with repeated use of the same drug, causing decreased responsiveness to that drug. Larger doses of the drug are required to produce the same level of response as was initially attained.

Tachyphylaxis—Rapidly developing tolerance occurring with repeated doses of the same drug. For example, repeated and excessive use of catecholamines leads to increased activity and concentration of catechol-O-methyltransferase (COMT) in the synaptic junction. This results in β_2 blockade; rebound bronchoconstriction may then occur.

Cumulation—Toxic conditions may occur within the body when the rate of elimination of a drug is slower than the rate of administration (e.g., as in renal failure). The desired effect is a steady state: drug in equals drug out.

Age—Drug dosage is a factor of body weight and surface area, which must be adjusted for children and the elderly.

Drug allergies—Hypersensitivity to a drug may cause an anaphylactic reaction.

Patient noncompliance—The desired effects may not be noted if the patient refuses to comply with the dosing regimen.

Pregnancy—Administering drugs that cross the placental barrier may be harmful and cause teratogenic effects to the fetus owing to an incomplete and immature enzyme system.

5 Therapeutic Evaluation and Preparation of Medicines

Therapeutic maintenance includes supportive care of the patient and the proficient use of pharmacologic agents. The practitioner must have a thorough knowledge of respiratory drug action, interaction, and effects before skillfully administering and evaluating these drugs.

Objectives

1. Define and describe subjective data, objective data, assessment, and plan of action as it pertains to drug evaluation.
2. Interrelate the pharmacological assessment questions to the type of drug, dosage, administration, etc.
3. Specify the rules for good charting.
4. List the precautions taken when administering medications.
5. Name the most commonly used medication syringes. List the units in which the syringe scales are calibrated.
6. Compare/contrast the two methods in which medications may be "drawn up" by using syringes.
7. Describe the medicine cup, list the units found on the medicine cup, and identify how the dosage is read.
8. Identify the calibrated dropper and the special precautions observed when using the calibrated dropper.
9. Explain the unit dose method of drug administration and the advantages pertaining to the unit dose.

THE FOUR PARTS OF THERAPEUTIC EVALUATION

Evaluation of drug therapy is the process of determining the effectiveness of drug action. It is an exceedingly important step in identifying the particular needs of a patient. The evaluation is carried out purposefully and in an organized way. Four basic methods of collecting data for evaluation need to be employed by the practitioner: (*a*) subjective feelings of the patient, (*b*) observation and examination of the patient, (*c*) assessment of the patient and of the data collected, and (*d*) review of data and reports to determine the course of drug therapy. These methods are collectively termed SOAP, for subjective, objective, assessment, and plan.

Subjective

Subjective data is discernible only to the person affected and can only be verified by the person involved. After the administration of respiratory therapeutics, a patient's subjective feeling of comfort, relief of bronchospasm, and well-being is probably the most valuable tool in determining the effectiveness of therapy.

Objective

Objective data is that which is detectable by the practitioner or can be tested using acceptable standards. Overt data refers to something observed. Before, during, and after the administration of respiratory drugs, the practitioner must note pulse, respirations, auscultatory findings, and the volume of sputum production. Any noticeable improvement of the above may lead to a positive evaluation of the effectiveness of drug action.

Assessment

Assessment is the systematic collection of data and then the allocation of a meaning to the data. Data may be collected by observation, by interviewing, by physical examination, or by implementing specific tests that act as guidelines to determine the effectiveness of drug therapy. Bedside pulmonary function studies such as vital capacity, peak flow, and FEV_1 are completed before and after bronchodilator therapy to evaluate and document the extent of improvement. Monitoring arterial blood gas parameters and chest x-rays are also useful in assessing the effectiveness of drug action. Basic pharmacological assessment questions (Table 5.1) are also useful in the assessment of and the evaluation of drug therapy and drug effectiveness.

Table 5.1.
Pharmacological Assessment Questions[a]

Rationale for use	Why is the patient receiving this drug? Which problem is it intended to treat? (e.g., infection, bronchoconstriction, mucus retention)
Dosage	Is the ordered dosage appropriate?
Administration	Is the mode of administration appropriate? (e.g., intravenous, oral, inhalation)
Effects	Does the drug produce the desired action and effects? Is there observed improvement? Would another drug or dosage be more effective?
Side effects	Are side effects present? If so, have they been minimized to a tolerable level? Would another drug produce less adverse effects, yet promote the same effectiveness?
Patient compliance	Does the patient feel he or she is benefiting from drug therapy and thereby complying with the regimen?

[a]Adapted from Kersten L. *Comprehensive Respiratory Nursing*. Philadelphia: WB Saunders, 1989. Used with permission.

Plan

All other steps in the evaluation of drug therapy depend on the collection of data, which needs to be complete, relevant, and carefully recorded. A plan of action is necessary to implement, modify, or alter the course of drug therapy. The practitioner must review on a daily basis the course of drug therapy pertaining to a particular patient. After careful review and assessment of the data available, the practitioner may intelligently recommend any modifications that may be necessary for the progress of the patient. In many cases, the physician relies heavily on the information and recommendations relayed to him or her by the practitioner.

RULES FOR GOOD CHARTING

Most practitioners give medications to patients more often than any other single task. Before administering and charting any drug, make certain the "five rights" are observed: give the *right dose* of the *right medication* to the *right patient* at the *right time* by the *right route*. To prevent errors and ensure safe administration, always check the physician's medical orders for date, drug, dosage, route, and frequency.

The primary purpose of charting is to ensure continuity of patient care.

Keeping well constructed, accurate, and complete notes not only ensures this continuity of care and protects your patient, but also protects you from any forms of malpractice or negligence litigation if you are ever brought to court. Your notes serve as a legal document and should thus comply with the following guidelines for good charting:

1. Conform to hospital policy regarding notes, and follow up that policy with sound professional judgment. Record only on the proper forms supplied.
2. Enter the date and time before each note. Sign each note with your first initial, last name, and your title (e.g., R.N., C.R.T.T., R.R.T., etc.)
3. Never erase or write between the lines. If a mistake is made, draw a line through it, write "error" and sign your initials.
4. Record on every line in chronological order. Draw a line through any unused or half-used lines before signing your name.
5. Don't let anyone else chart or sign for the care you have given. Don't chart or sign for any care others have given.
6. Don't generalize in your charting; be specific and exclude any bias from your charting.
7. Document any discussions of questionable medical orders and the physician's directives to the order and the actions you took.
8. Record your patient assessment before and after therapy.
9. Above all, maintain accurate records—it is well worth the time and effort.

PREPARATION OF MEDICINES

There are several methods to prepare or "draw up" medications. This section focuses on the primary systems.

Syringes

Figure 5.1 shows the three types of syringes most commonly used for medication preparation. The tuberculin syringe (1-cc dosage), the 3-cc syringe, and the 6-cc syringe have double calibrated scales that measure dosages in cc on one side and minims on the other side.

Two methods are available for drawing up medications with syringes. The *single syringe method* uses one syringe for drug administration. This system is preferred when only one agent is required. However, it may also be used when an active ingredient (e.g., albuterol) and a diluent (e.g., normal saline) are needed. Both the active ingredient and diluent are drawn into the syringe in proper proportions (e.g., 0.5 ml albuterol plus 2.5 ml normal saline). Disadvantages to this system include possible cross-contamination and inaccurate dosage when two agents are mixed in one syringe.

The *double or separate syringe method* uses two syringes for drug administration. The active ingredient is drawn into one syringe while the diluent is drawn into another separate syringe. This allows for accuracy of drug dosage while eliminating cross-contamination of the agents used. This is the preferred method when two or more agents are used.

Medicine Cup

The medicine cup is a small plastic 30-cc cup (Fig. 5.2) that has the following graduations:

teaspoons (tsp)	ounces (oz)
tablespoons (tbs)	drams
dessertspoons (dssp)	milliliters (ml)
	cubic centimeters (cc)

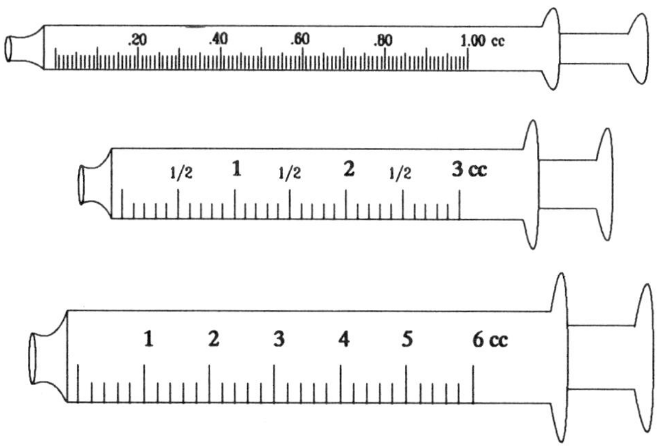

Figure 5.1. Commonly used medication syringes.

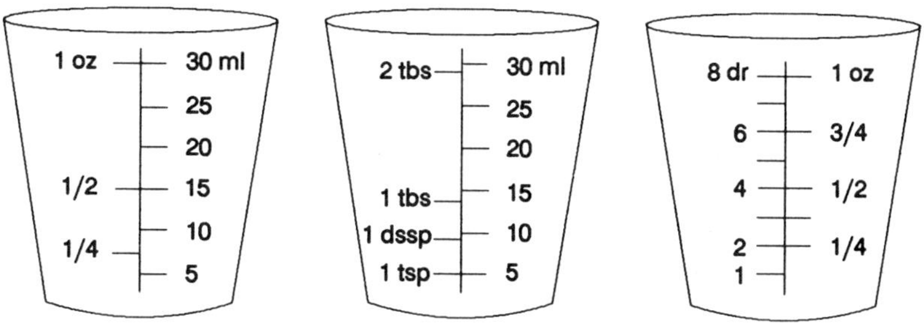

Figure 5.2. Commonly used medicine cups with various graduations.

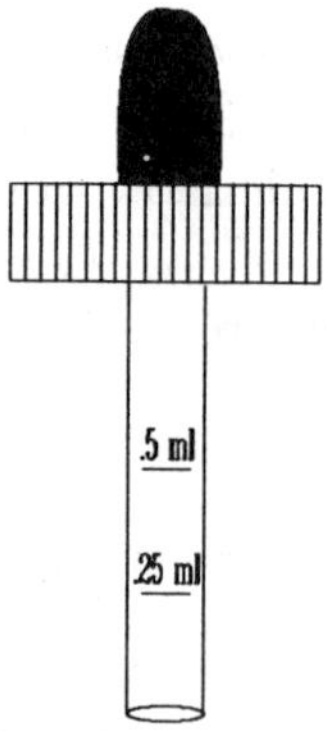

Figure 5.3. The calibrated dropper.

Measurements of teaspoons, tablespoons, and dessertspoons are in the household measuring system; measurements of ounces and drams are apothecary measures, and milliliters and cubic centimeters are of the metric system.

The reading of the dose must be made at the lowest point of the meniscus and observed at eye level. If more than one agent is used, careful consideration of dosage dilution and accuracy must be realized. Cross-contamination of vials is prevented if agents are drawn up separately then added to the measuring cup, or if they are poured separately into the cup.

Calibrated Dropper

Certain drugs are supplied with a calibrated dropper (Fig. 5.3). Graduations may be milliliters, cubic centimeters, teaspoons, or ounces. Careful consideration must be given to eliminate air bubbles and excess solution. Drug manufacturers have specific calibration guidelines for a particular drug, therefore substituting a medicine dropper to use with a drug other than the one recommended may result in inaccurate dosage.

Unit Dose

The unit dose method provides a one-time-use, premeasured dosage placed in a container (usually a vial or ampul). The container may contain the active ingredient alone or the active ingredient mixed with a diluent. Medication errors and drug waste are eliminated, which results in safe administration and lower costs for the patient.

6 Mathematics of Drugs and Solutions

One of the more difficult areas of drug therapy for practitioners is the mathematics of drugs and solutions. The comprehension and application of mathematical concepts as applied to the administration of drugs and solutions is of utmost importance to the practitioner, as calculations must be made and accuracy is essential.

Objectives

1. Name and describe the systems of measurement, their symbols and abbreviations, and any special considerations for use. Apply the conversions of equivalents within and between the metric, the apothecary, and the household methods.
2. Define the terms applied to solutions.
3. Convert percentage strength to a ratio (for example; a 5% solution is 5 g/100 ml, which is a 1:20 ratio).
4. Convert a given amount of grams/100 ml to mg/ml (for example; 5 g/100 ml equals 5000 mg/100 ml, which is 50 mg/ml).
5. When given a drug dosage problem, provide an appropriate equation to solve for an unknown variable. The unknown variable may be
   - the percentage strength,
   - the solute,
   - the total solution amount, or
   - the desired dosage needed for administration.
6. Identify the rules of drug dosage that apply to children and infants.
7. Calculate and solve the problems listed in the drug calculation exercise.

METHODS OF MEASUREMENT

The Metric System

The metric system—also called the decimal system—is a method of weights and measures using multiples and fractions of 10. Denominations may be changed by simply moving the decimal point. The metric system is the most commonly used system of measurement owing to its accuracy and uniformity.

The unit of length in this system is the meter (hence "metric"). The units applied to weight (i.e., the kilogram, the gram, and the milligram) and the units applied to volume (i.e., the liter and the milliliter or the cubic centimeter) are used to measure medications.

Primary Units

METER (M, m)	unit of LENGTH
GRAM (g, gm, Gm)	unit of WEIGHT
LITER (L, l)	unit of VOLUME

Latin prefixes are designated to express quantities *less* than a meter, a gram, or a liter.

Unit	Meaning	Written As
nano (n)	10^{-9}	0.000000001
micro (μ)	10^{-6}	0.000001
milli (m)	10^{-3}	0.001
centi (c)	10^{-2}	0.01
deci (d)	10^{-1}	0.1

For all quantities less than one, decimal fractions are used (i.e., 0.5 g, 0.1 g)

Greek prefixes are designated to express quantities *greater* than a meter, a gram, or a liter.

Unit	Meaning	Written As
kilo (k)	10^3	1000
hecto (h)	10^2	100
deca (da)	10	10
meter, gram, liter	1	1

Summary

Weight		Volume	
kilogram (kg)	$g \times 10^3$	kiloliter (kl)	$L \times 10^3$
hectogram (hg)	$g \times 10^2$	hectoliter (hl)	$L \times 10^2$
decagram (dag)	$g \times 10$	decaliter (dal)	$L \times 10$

gram (g, gm, Gm)	1	liter (L, l)	1
decigram (dg)	$g \times 10^{-1}$	deciliter (dl)	$L \times 10^{-1}$
centigram (cg)	$g \times 10^{-2}$	centiliter (cl)	$L \times 10^{-2}$
milligram (mg)	$g \times 10^{-3}$	milliliter (ml)	$L \times 10^{-3}$
microgram (μg)	$g \times 10^{-6}$	microliter (μl)	$L \times 10^{-6}$
nanogram (ng)	$g \times 10^{-9}$	nanoliter (nl)	$L \times 10^{-9}$

Equivalents within the Metric System

Weight	Volume
1 gram = 1000 mg	1 liter = 1000 ml*
= 100 cg	= 100 cl
= 10 dg	= 10 dl
= 0.1 dag	= 0.1 dal
= 0.01 hg	= 0.01 hl
= 0.001 kg	= 0.001 kl

*ml is frequently written as cc (cubic centimeter). Both terms represent 1/1000 of a liter. For general purposes, 1 ml = 1 cc and weighs 1 g (water at 4°C)

Helpful Hints

1. 10 times 1 unit = the next higher unit
   Example: 10 × 1 mg = 1 cg
   10 × 1 cg = 1 dg
   10 × 1 dg = 1 g
2. Placing the decimal point one place to the right multiplies its value by 10.
   Example: 0.001 × 10 = 0.01
3. Placing the decimal point one place to the left divides its value by 10.
   Example: 0.001/10 = 0.0001

The Apothecary System

The apothecary system is an ancient English method that is being replaced by the metric system. However, some hospitals and physicians still use this system.

Apothecary Weight

The units for weighing solids are (from smallest to largest):

grain (gr)
scruple (℈)
dram (ʒ)
ounce (℥, oz)
pound (lb)

In apothecary weight, 12 ounces equal 1 pound, whereas in avoirdupois weight 16 ounces equal 1 pound.

Apothecary Volume

The units for measuring volume are (from smallest to largest):

minim (♏)
fluidram (f ʒ)
fluidounce (f ℥)
pint (pt)
quart (qt)
gallon (gal)

Equivalents within the Apothecary System

Weight		Volume	
20 grains	= 1 scruple	60 minims*	= 1 fluidram
3 scruples	= 1 dram	8 fluidrams	= 1 fluidounce
8 drams	= 1 ounce	16 fluidounces	= 1 pint
12 ounces	= 1 pound	2 pints	= 1 quart
		4 quarts	= 1 gallon

*One minim *is almost equal to one drop.* A minim is measured with a minim glass and a drop is measured with a medicine dropper. For accuracy, if a drug is prescribed in minims, it is best to measure it in minims, not drops.

Symbols and Abbreviations

Lowercase Roman numerals and fractions express quantities in the apothecary system. When a symbol or abbreviation of a unit is used, the symbol or abbreviation is expressed first, followed by the quantity, written either in Roman numerals or as a fraction.

For example, if the quantity is 1 or greater, Roman numerals are used:

2 drams is ʒ ii
6 grains is gr vi

If the quantity is less than 1, fractions are used:

¼ ounce is ℥ ¼ or oz ¼
¾ grain is gr ¾

An exception to the rule is the fraction ½, which has its own symbol, $\overline{ss}$. Therefore, an order for ½ grain may be written as gr $\overline{ss}$.

5½ ounces is ℥ v$\overline{ss}$
7½ grains is gr vii$\overline{ss}$

Some Commonly Used Symbols and Lowercase Roman Numerals

$\overline{ss}$ = ½	iii = 3	vi = 6	ix = 9
i = 1	iv = 4	vii = 7	x = 10
ii = 2	v = 5	viii = 8	xv = 15

Approximate Conversion Equivalents*

	Metric	Apothecary
Weight	60 milligrams	1 grain
	1 gram (1000 mg)	15 grains
Volume	1 ml	16 minims
	30 ml	1 fluidounce
	500 ml	1 pint
	1000 ml	1 quart

*For a complete list of conversion equivalents, refer to Appendix A.

The Household System

The household system of measurement is the least accurate method of weights and measures and contains only approximate equivalents. Therefore, it is not advisable to substitute household equivalents for medication prescribed by physicians. The household system is used only when it is impractical to measure doses by other systems. This system is based on cooking utensils such as the teaspoon and tablespoon and is commonly used in everyday home situations.

Household Measurements

60 drops (gtt)	= 1 teaspoon (t)	2 cups	= 1 pint (pt)
3 teaspoonfuls	= 1 tablespoon (T)	2 pints	= 1 quart (qt)
2 tablespoonfuls	= 1 fluidounce (oz)	1 quart	= 4 cups
8 fluidounces	= 1 glassful	4 quarts	= 1 gallon (gal)
16 ounces (dry measure)	= 1 pound		

Approximate Conversion Equivalents

Metric	Apothecary	Household
0.06 ml	1 minim	1 drop
1 ml	16 minims	16 drops
4 or 5 ml	1 fluidram	1 teaspoon
15 ml	½ fluidounce	1 tablespoon
30 ml	1 fluidounce	2 tablespoons

240 ml (≈250 ml)	8 fluidounces	1 cup
473 ml (≈500 ml)	16 fluidounces	1 pint
946 ml (≈1,000 ml)	32 fluidounces	1 quart
3,785 ml	128 fluidounces	1 gallon

The Avoirdupois System

The avoirdupois method is a system of weight only and is mainly used in English-speaking countries. The avoirdupois and the apothecary systems contain the same terms, yet the grain is the only term that is an equal amount. The avoirdupois pound contains 16 ounces, while the apothecary pound contains 12 ounces.

Avoirdupois Measurements

437.5 grains = 1 ounce
16 ounces = 1 pound
7000 grains = 1 pound

Approximate Conversion Equivalents*

Metric	Avoirdupois
1 g	0.035274 ounce
28.3 g	1 ounce
454 g	1 pound
1 kg	2.2 pounds

*Note: All the above lists of equivalents are only *approximate*. Different sets of equivalents can be found in different texts.

CHEMICAL SOLUTIONS: DEFINITIONS AND TERMS

Solute: The substance dissolved in a solution (the active ingredient).

Solvent: The dissolving medium (the component in a solution present in the greatest amount).

Solution: A homogeneous mixture of one or more substances (solute) dissolved in a quantity of a dissolving medium (solvent).

Aqueous solution: A solution in which water is the dissolving medium.

Strength of a solution: Percentage of solute present in a solution, expressed as parts of solute in 100 parts solution.

Normal solution: A solution in which 1 liter contains 1 gram equivalent of the solute.

Buffer solution: A solution of a weak acid and its salt—maintains a constant pH.

Milliequivalent (mEq): Concentration of electrolytes in a certain volume (usually 1 liter) of solution.

Molar solution: A solution in which 1 mole (Avogadro's number) of the solute is dissolved in 1 liter.

Osmolar solution: Concentration of osmotically active particles in solution.

Isotonic, hypertonic, hypotonic solutions: See glossary of terms (Ch. 1) and Inhalational Mucolytic Agents (Ch. 15).

DRUG DOSAGE CALCULATIONS

Solutions Whose Strength Is Expressed in Percentage

Three types of percentage preparations exist:

Weight-to-weight (W/W): the amount (grams of active ingredient) in 100 grams of a mixture.

$$W/W\% = \frac{\text{grams (solute)}}{\text{100 grams (solution)}} \times 100$$

Example: 1% contains 1 g/100 g

Weight-to-Volume (W/V): the amount (grams of active ingredient) in 100 milliliters of a mixture.

$$W/V\% = \frac{\text{grams (solute)}}{\text{100 milliliters (solution)}} \times 100$$

Example: 5% contains 5 g/100 ml

Prescription usage favors weight-to-volume percentage solutions. When a ratio or percent is given of a drug strength it is understood to be g:ml unless otherwise stated.

Volume-to-Volume (V/V): the amount (milliliters of active ingredient) in 100 milliliters of a mixture.

$$V/V\% = \frac{\text{milliliters (solute)}}{\text{100 milliliters (solution)}} \times 100$$

Example: 0.1% contains 0.1 ml/100 ml

Solutions Whose Strength Is Expressed in Ratio

A ratio designates the relation between the solute and the solvent and is usually expressed in g:ml. However, "ratio by simple parts" still exists. For example, a physician may order Bronkosol 1:8, which means one part drug to eight parts diluent. This type of drug order does not give the actual dosage amount, although milliliters is assumed. Your knowledge of correct dosage when interpreting this type of order is essential. The dosage range for Bronkosol 1% is 0.25 to 0.5 ml diluted with normal saline, therefore you would not give more than this.

Ratio by g:ml

Examples:

A physician has written orders for your patient to receive Isuprel 1:200 by nebulization.

Isuprel 1:200 is expressed as 1g:200 ml.

Calculating the percentage strength gives:

$$W/V\% = \text{solute/total solution} \times 100 = 1/200 \times 100 = 0.5\%$$

Isuprel 1:200 has a strength of 0.5%.

A 1:100 solute to solvent ratio (1 g:100 ml) has a strength of 1%:

$$1/100 \times 100 = 1\%$$

Ratio by mg:ml

Remember: 1000 mg = 1 g

Isuprel 1:200 = 1 g:200 ml = 1000 mg:200 ml = 5 mg:ml or 5 mg.

Isuprel 1:200 has a strength of 0.5% and contains 5 mg. (or 0.005 g)

1:100 = 1 g:100 ml = 1000 mg:100 ml = 10 mg:ml or 10 mg.

1:100 has a strength of 1% and contains 10 mg.

Percentage and Ratios of Solutions
Weight to Volume

Ratio	Percentage (%)	g/ml	mg/ml
1:1000	0.1	0.001	1
1:500	0.2	0.002	2
1:200	0.5	0.005	5
1:100	1	0.01	10
1:20	5	0.05	50
1:10	10	0.1	100
1:5	20	0.2	200
1:1	100	1	1000

Percentage and Ratio Calculations

$$\text{Percent strength (in decimals)} = \frac{\text{solute (g or ml)}}{\text{total solution (ml)}}$$

This equation provides three variables:

a. If solute amount and total solution amount are known, solve for strength.
b. If total solution amount and strength are given, solve for solute.
c. If solute and strength are given, solve for total amount.

Rules:

1. If a ratio is given (e.g., 1:200) it must be converted to g/ml (e.g., 1 g:200 ml = 0.005 g/ml.
2. Solute (if given in milligrams) must be converted to grams.

Examples:

1a. What is the percentage strength of a solution which contains 5 g of drug to 100 ml of solution?
x = percent
5 g = solute
100 ml = total amount

$$x = 5 \text{ g}/100 \text{ ml} = 0.05\ (\times\ 100) = 5\%$$

1b. Express the ratio in milligrams.

$$5 \text{ g}:100 \text{ ml} = 5000 \text{ mg}:100 \text{ ml} = 50 \text{ mg}$$

2. How many milligrams are there in 4 ml 1:100 epinephrine?
x = amount of solute
4 ml = total amount
strength = 1:100 = 0.01 g/ml

$$0.01 = x/4$$
$$0.01 \times 4 = x = .04 \text{ g}$$
$$0.04 \text{ g} = 40 \text{ mg}$$

3. A physician orders Isuprel 1:200, 2 mg to be administered to your patient diluted with 2.5 cc normal saline. What is the amount of Isuprel you will give to your patient?
x = total amount
solute = 2 mg = 0.002 g

$$\text{strength} = 1:200 = 0.005 \text{ g/ml}$$
$$0.005 = 0.002/x$$
$$0.002/0.005 = x = 0.4 \text{ ml}$$

Another type of percentage equation is to apply the known terms to a ratio or proportion.

$$A:B::C:D \text{ or } A/B = C/D$$

A and D (the first and fourth terms) are the "extremes"
B and C (the second and third terms) are the "means"
The product of the means equals the product of the extremes.

Example:

$$2:3::4:6 \text{ or } 2/3 = 4/6$$
$$2 \times 6 = 3 \times 4$$

To express the percentage ratio:

$$\text{Desired \%} : \text{Have \%} :: \text{Small quantity} : \text{Large quantity}$$

or

$$\frac{\text{Desired \%}}{\text{Have \%}} = \frac{\text{Small quantity before dilution}}{\text{Large quantity after dilution}}$$

Example: Mucomyst is prepared in 10% and 20% solutions. You have on hand a 20% Mucomyst solution. The physician orders 8 ml of 10% Mucomyst to be administered by nebulization. How many ml of the 20% solution are needed to prepare a 10% solution?

Desired % = 10
Have % = 20
Small quantity before dilution = x
Large quantity after dilution = 8 ml

$$10/20 = x/8$$
$$10 \times 8 = 20x$$
$$80/20 = x = 4$$

4 ml of the 20% Mucomyst solution added with 4 ml of normal saline will give your patient 8 ml of a 10% Mucomyst solution.

Example: Prepare a 3-ml dose of isoetharine 0.2% from a stock solution containing 1% isoetharine.

Desired % = 0.2
Have % = 1
Small quantity before dilution = x
Large quantity after dilution = 3 ml

$$0.2/1 = x/3$$
$$0.2 \times 3 = 1x$$
$$0.6 = x$$

0.6 ml of 1% isoetharine added to 2.4 ml of normal saline will give 3 ml of 0.2% isoetharine.

Calculating Dosages from Stock Solutions, Tablets, Capsules, and Liquids

Within the Same System

This involves a two-step process:

1. Convert the amount to be given into a common unit with the amount of the drug on hand.
2. Set up a ratio.

Example: A physician orders 1 g ampicillin to be administered to your patient. You have on hand 250-mg ampicillin capsules.

1. Convert grams to milligrams: 1 g = 1000 mg
2. Set up a ratio:

$$\overset{\textit{Unknown}}{\frac{\text{desired dosage}}{\text{desired amount}}} = \overset{\textit{Known}}{\frac{\text{original strength}}{\text{amount supplied}}}$$

In the above example there are three known terms: 250 mg (original strength) per capsule (amount supplied), total dosage to be administered 1000 mg (1 g) (desired dosage).

The unknown term is how many capsules should be given (desired amount).

$$1000/x = 250/1$$
$$1000 = 250x$$
$$1000/250 = x = 4$$

You will give your patient 4 capsules for a dose of 1 g.

From One System to Another

This involves the same two-step process:

Example: A physician orders gr i$\overline{\text{ss}}$ of a drug to be administered. Stock tablets on hand contain 0.2 g each.

1. Convert the amount to be given into a common unit with the amount of the drug on hand.

   Referring to the table of equivalents: 1 gram = 15 grains.
   How many grains are in each tablet?

$$0.2 \text{ gram}:? \text{ grains}::1 \text{ gram}:15 \text{ grains}$$
$$0.2/x = 1/15$$
$$0.2 \times 15 = x = 3$$

There are 3 grains in each tablet.

2. Set up a ratio:

$$\begin{array}{ccc} \textit{Unknown} & & \textit{Known} \\ \dfrac{\text{desired dosage}}{\text{desired amount}} & = & \dfrac{\text{original strength}}{\text{amount supplied}} \end{array}$$

The three known terms are: dosage is 1.5 grains (desired dosage). There are 3 grains (original strength) per tablet (amount supplied).
The unknown term is how many tablets should be given (desired amount).

$$1.5/x = 3/1$$
$$1.5 = 3x$$
$$1.5/3 = x = 0.5$$

You will give your patient ½ tablet.

To Give Units

Some drugs are supplied in ampules or vials that contain a specific number of units per cc of solution.
Example: An ampule of Tetanus antitoxin contains "1500 U per cc." How much of the solution would you give if the physician has ordered a total dose of 1000 units?

$$\frac{\text{desired dosage}}{\text{desired amount}} = \frac{\text{original strength}}{\text{amount supplied}}$$

$$\frac{1000 \text{ U}}{(x) \text{ cc}} = \frac{1500 \text{ U}}{1 \text{ cc}}$$

$$1000 = 1500x$$
$$1000/1500 = x = 0.67 \text{ or } 2/3$$

You will give ⅔ cc of the antitoxin.

DOSAGE FOR CHILDREN AND INFANTS

Dosages of drugs for children and infants are reduced proportionately to the age or weight of the child. Various rules apply.

Young's Rule (for children 2–12 years)

$$\text{Child's dose} = \frac{\text{age in years}}{\text{age in years} + 12} \times \text{adult dose}$$

Clark's Rule

$$\text{Child's dose} = \frac{\text{weight in pounds}}{150} \times \text{adult dose}$$

Fried's Rule (children <2 years)

$$\text{Child's dose} = \frac{\text{age in months}}{150} \times \text{adult dose}$$

Cowling's Rule

$$\text{Child's dose} = \frac{\text{age next birthday}}{24} \times \text{adult dose}$$

These rules are intended to serve as an approximate guide only. Other factors such as physiologic and pathologic conditions may also regulate the dose of a drug.

EXERCISE IN DRUG DOSAGE CALCULATION

1. A patient with severe myasthenia gravis is to receive Mestinon syrup 0.36 g. The stock dosage on hand is 60 mg/5 ml. How many milliliters will the patient receive? Convert this amount to ounces.
2. How many milligrams are in 3 ml of 1:100 epinephrine?
3. A patient is to receive 20 mg of prednisone. Each tablet contains 5 mg. How many tablets will you administer?
4. A patient is to receive aspirin gr x. The tablets on hand are 0.33 g per tablet. How many tablets will you give?
5. Penicillin 750,000 units is to be given. The stock on hand contains 300,000 units per cc. How many cc will you administer?
6. A 100-mg dose is needed from a drug containing 75 mg/cc. How many cc are needed?

7. You have on hand epinephrine 1:100. How many milliliters of this solution contain 30 mg of epinephrine?

8. If a drug contains 5% strength, how many mg of active ingredient are in 40 ml of the solution?

9. You have a solution containing 500 mg/cc. You are to administer 400 mg. How much solution will you give?

10. You have on hand a 10% solution. Prepare 4 ml at 8% strength.

Conversions

11. 75 mg = _____ grains
12. 20 ml = _____ cc
13. 12 gtt = _____ ml
14. 20 oz = _____ ml
15. 0.5 g = _____ grains
16. 8 drams = _____ ml
17. 0.2 ml = _____ minims
18. gr vii = _____
19. ʒ drams ix$\overline{ss}$ = _____
20. ℥ ounce i = _____

ANSWERS

1. 0.36 g/x = 0.06 g/5 ml
   0.36 × 5 = 0.06(x)
   x = 30 ml
   30 ml = 1 ounce
2. 0.01 = x/3 ml
   x = 0.01 × 3
   = 0.03 g
   0.03 g = 30 mg
3. 20 mg/x = 5 mg/1 tablet
   20 = 5(x)
   x = 4 tablets

4a. 1 gram = 15 grains
   0.33g/x = 1 g/15 grains
   0.33 × 15 = x
   4.95 grains = x

b. 10/x = 4.95/1
   10 = 4.95(x)
   x = 2 tablets

5. 750,000/x = 300,000/1
   750,000 = 300,000(x)
   x = 2.5 cc
6. 100 mg/x = 75 mg/1 cc
   100 = 75(x)
   x = 1.33 cc
7. 0.01 = 0.03 g/x(ml)
   0.01(x) = 0.03
   x = 3 ml
8. 0.05 = x(g)/40 ml
   0.05 × 40 = x
   x = 2 g
   2 g = 2000 mg

9. 400 mg/x = 500 mg/1 cc
   400 = 500(x)
   x = 0.8 cc
10. 8%/10% = x/4 ml
   8 × 4 = 10(x)
   32/10 = x = 3.2 ml
   3.2 ml of 10% solution plus 0.8 ml of normal saline gives 4 ml at 8% strength.
11. 60 mg = 1 grain
   75/x = 60/1
   75/60 = 1¼ grains
12. 1 ml = 1 cc
   20 ml = 20 cc
13. 16 gtt = 1 ml
   12/x = 16/1
   12/16 = 0.75 ml
14. 1 ounce = 30 ml
   20/x = 1/30
   20 × 30 = 600 ml
15. 1 gram = 15 grains
   0.5/x = 1/15
   0.5 × 15 = 7.5 grains
16. 8 drams = 1 oz = 30 ml
17. 1 ml = 16 minims
   x/0.2 = 16/1
   0.2 × 16 = 3.2 minims
18. 7 grains
19. 9½ drams
20. 1 ounce

Individual Pharmacologic Agents II

Chapters 7 through 20 present the specific pharmacologic agents. For consistency, each of the chapters is organized in the same manner and the objectives for these chapters are summarized as follows:

1. If included, discuss the preparatory review and how it relates to the drugs presented in the chapter.
2. Identify and discuss the mechanism of action, indications, and contraindications as they pertain to each specific drug category.
3. List the precautions, adverse reactions, and symptoms of overdose as they pertain to each specific drug category.
4. Identify and group each agent to its particular category or group.
5. List the appropriate dosage of each bronchodilator (it is essential for the cardiopulmonary practitioner to know the appropriate dosage of each bronchodilator and to have a general awareness of the proper dosages of critical care drugs and those drugs used during the resuscitation procedure).
6. List and identify any special applications, considerations as they pertain to a specific agent.

Note: All drug dosages presented in the following chapters are to be used as a general guideline only, not as absolute. Many factors play a vital role in determining the proper dosage for a certain patient. Chapters 2, 3, and 4 presented the various mechanisms that can alter or modify a drug's action and final effect. These same mechanisms also apply to a drug's dosage.

7 Cough and Cold Preparations

The tremendous variety of cough and cold remedies, available either over the counter or by prescription, do not cure the cold nor lessen its duration, but only serve to modify or relieve the symptoms present (nasal congestion, headache, fever, general malaise, cough, rhinorrhea). This chapter focuses on the four classes of drugs that work, either singly or in combination with each other, to lessen the severity of the cough, cold, or allergy symptoms.

The efficacy of some of these agents is questionable owing to the lack of objective studies. Many over-the-counter cold and cough remedies are used indiscriminantly, therefore their potential for abuse is high. Of utmost importance is the need to first treat the underlying *cause* of the cough or allergy.

The addition of other chemicals such as analgesics, anticholinergic agents, preservatives, caffeine, and alcohol is a common but questionable practice. Anticholinergics (such as atropine or methscopolamine) are included for their drying effects on mucosal secretions; however, this may lead to mucus plugging or airway obstruction. Caffeine is included in some preparations for CNS stimulation to counteract the effects of antihistamine depression. Analgesics (acetaminophen, aspirin, sodium salicylate) are added for symptoms of headache, fever, and muscle aches and pain. Some preparations contain considerable alcohol levels. When using these combinations it is necessary to consider whether each ingredient is applicable to the symptoms or condition present, or whether a particular ingredient is even beneficial. Since there are a variety of cough and cold preparations available, it allows one to be very selective.

NASAL DECONGESTANTS

MECHANISM OF ACTION AND INDICATIONS FOR USE:

Decongestants are sympathomimetic amines with primary α-receptor action. Activation of the α receptor sites elicits marked vasoconstriction, which in turn causes shrinkage of the nasal mucosa, thereby relieving membrane congestion. Decongestants administered topically to swollen membranes or systemically via the oral route are useful for the treatment of mucosal congestion accompanying hay fever, allergic rhinitis, acute coryza, sinusitis, and other respiratory conditions.

CONTRAINDICATIONS:

Hypersensitivity to sympathomimetic amines, severe hypertension, coronary artery disease, nursing mothers. Monoamine oxidase inhibitor (MAO) therapy.

PRECAUTIONS:

1. Excessive topical use may result in systemic effects resulting in nervousness, dizziness, or sleeplessness.
2. Rebound congestion (hyperemia, edema of mucosa) may occur following topical administration once the vasoconstrictive effects recede.
3. Use topical administration of decongestants only in acute states, and no longer than 3 to 5 days.

ADVERSE REACTIONS:

Cardiovascular: Palpitations, tachycardia, arrhythmias, cardiovascular collapse.

CNS: Fear, anxiety, headache, restlessness, lightheadedness, dizziness, drowsiness, tremor, insomnia, hallucinations, convulsions, CNS depression.

GI: Nausea, vomiting, anorexia.

GU: Urinary retention, dysuria.

Topical administration: Burning, stinging, sneezing, dryness, mucosal irritation, rebound congestion.

Miscellaneous: Respiratory difficulties, sweating, pallor.

OVERDOSAGE:

CNS depression accompanied by hypertension, bradycardia, and rebound hypotension. Somnolence, sedation, or deep coma may also occur. Treatment consists of supportive care and early intervention with gastric lavage following oral overdose.

Tables 7.1 and 7.2 list the nasal decongestants.

Table 7.1.
Nasal Decongestants for Adults

Decongestant	Route[a]	Dosage[b]
Phenylpropanolamine HCl (Propagest, Rhindecon)	O O-SR	25 mg q 4 hr 75 mg q 12 hr
Pseudoephedrine HCl (Genaphed Tablets, Halofed, Sudafed, Sudrin, Cenafed, Neofed, Novafed)	O O-SR	60 mg q 6 hr 120 mg q 12 hr
Phenylephrine HCl (Neo-Synephrine, Alconefrin, Rhinall, Doktors, Nostril, Sinex)	T	1 to 2 sprays or drops q 3 to 4 hr
Epinephrine HCl (Adrenalin Chloride)	T	up to 1 ml/15 min
Ephedrine (Vatronol Nose Drops, Efedron Nasal)	T	2 to 3 drops q 4 hr
Desoxyephedrine (Vicks Inhaler)	T	50-mg inhaler
Naphazoline HCl (Privine)	T	2 drops q 3 hr
Tetrahydrozoline HCl (Tyzine)	T	2 to 4 drops q 3 hr
Oxymetazoline HCl (Afrin, Allerest, Coricidin, Duration, Dristan, Sinarest)	T	2 to 3 drops twice daily
Xylometazoline HCl (Otrivin)	T	2 to 3 drops q 8 to 10 hr
Propylhexedrine (Benzedrex)	T	250-mg inhaler

[a]Route: O, oral; O-SR, oral - sustained release; T, topical.
[b]Usual adult oral dose.

Table 7.2.
Pediatric Nasal Decongestants

Decongestant	Dosage
Pseudoephedrine HCl	
Sudafed	6–12 yr: 30 mg q 6 hr
Novafed	2–5 yr: 15 mg q 6 hr
Halofed	4 m–2 yr: 3.75 mg q 4 to 6 hr
PediaCare Infants' Cold Relief	
Phenylephrine HCl	
Neo-Synephrine	>6 yr: 0.25%; 2 sprays each nostril q 3 to 4 hr
St. Joseph Measured Dose Nasal Decongestant	infants: 0.125%, 0.2%; 1 drop each nostril q 2 to 4 hr
Tetrahydrozoline HCl	
Tyzine Pediatric Drops	2–6 yr: 2 to 3 drops of 0.05% solution in each nostril q 4 to 6 hr
Oxymetazoline HCl	
Afrin Children's Nose Drops	2–5 yr: 0.025%; 2 to 3 drops each nostril bid
Neo-Synephrine 12 Hour Children's Drops	
Xylometazoline HCl	
Neo-Synephrine II Long Acting Children's Nose Drops	2–12 yr: 0.05%; 2 or 3 drops each nostril q 8 to 10 hr
Otrivin Pediatric Nasal Drops	

ANTIHISTAMINES

Review of Histamine Action and Effects (see also Chapters 2 and 13)

Histamine is a vasoactive substance found in most body tissues (the highest concentration being in the lungs, skin, and stomach) and exists in bound form within subcellular granules of the mast cell. High concentrations of histamine are also located within the basophil blood cell. Various physical and chemical stimuli (including drugs and antigen-antibody reactions) mediate the release of histamine from the mast cell. Once histamine is released from the mast cell, a series of pathological reactions are triggered that range from mild itching to shock and death.

Released histamine acts on and binds to two separate and distinct receptors: H_1 and H_2. Activation of H_1 receptors causes increased capillary permeability and formation of edema and wheal, and induces contraction of bronchiolar and gastrointestinal smooth muscle, whereas activation of H_2 receptors causes cardiac acceleration (increased contractility and rate) and increased gastric acid production.

MECHANISM OF ACTION AND INDICATIONS FOR USE:

Antihistamines competitively block histamine at the H_1 receptor sites, thereby antagonizing the pharmacological effects histamine produces at the H_1 receptor. Antihistamines have neglible influence on H_2 receptors. The ability of antihistamines to block histamine action depends on both the concentration of histamine present and the concentration of the drug present. Antihistamines also exhibit anticholinergic (drying), antipruritic, sedative, and antiemetic effects.

Antihistamines are indicated for use in the relief of symptoms accompanying allergic rhinitis, vasomotor rhinitis, allergic conjunctivitis, angioedema, uncomplicated urticaria, and allergic reactions to blood or plasma, and also as an adjunctive therapy in anaphylactic reactions. Antihistamines with potent sedative effects are also used as nonprescription sleep aids, and those with antiemetic effects are used to treat nausea, vomiting, and motion sickness.

CONTRAINDICATIONS:

Antihistamine hypersensitivity, patients receiving monoamine oxidase (MAO) therapy. Not to be used in newborns, premature infants, or nursing mothers.

PRECAUTIONS:

1. Antihistamines are generally not indicated to treat lower respiratory tract symptoms owing to the antihistamines' anticholinergic (drying) effect, which may precipitate thickening of mucus secretions and hinder expectoration.
2. Patients must observe caution when driving or operating machinery, which require alertness.
3. Use phenothiazines with caution in patients with cardiovascular disease, liver impairment, or ulcer disease, (owing to cholestasia) also in children with history of sleep apnea, Reye's syndrome, or family history of sudden infant death syndrome (SIDS) (owing to diminished mental alertness).
4. Use with caution in the elderly—may cause dizziness, sedation, syncope, hypotension, or confusion.
5. Usage in pregnancy—use only if acutely indicated (antihistamines may cause harm to the fetus.) Especially not to be used during the third trimester.

6. Do not use with alcohol and other CNS depressants—additive effects are noted.
7. May cause GI upset—antihistamines should be taken with food.

ADVERSE REACTIONS:

Cardiovascular: Arrhythmias, hypertension, hypotension (elderly), palpitations, tachycardia.

CNS: Most frequent: drowsiness, sedation, dizziness, disturbed coordination, headache.

GI: Epigastric distress, nausea, vomiting.

GU: Urinary frequency, dysuria, urinary retention, impotence.

Pulmonary: Thickening of bronchial secretions, chest tightness, nasal congestion.

Miscellaneous: Tingling, heaviness and weakness of the hands, urticaria, rash, anaphylactic shock.

OVERDOSAGE:

Effects vary from CNS depression to CNS stimulation, cardiovascular collapse, and death. Treatment consists of supportive measures and early intervention with gastric lavage or the induction of vomiting. To minimize absorption administer activated charcoal following lavage.

There are five specific groups of compounds that constitute the antihistamines:

Alkylamines: Useful and effective at low doses and practical for daytime use. This group of antihistamines may cause either CNS stimulation (excitation) or CNS depression (sedation).

Ethanolamines: Gastrointestinal effects are minimal; however, ethanolamines have the highest incidence of drowsiness. Most of these agents are available by prescription only.

Ethylenediamines: Pyrilamine—high incidence of GI upset; may cause either moderate drowsiness or excitability and hyperirritability. Tripelennamine—low incidence of side effects; most frequent are drowsiness and dry mouth.

Phenothiazines: Strong CNS depressant effects; may suppress the cough reflex and obscure symptoms of intestinal obstruction, brain tumor, overdosage of toxic drugs.

Piperidines: Available by prescription only; may cause drowsiness and dryness of mouth.

Tables 7.3 and 7.4 list the antihistamines.

Table 7.3.
Antihistamines for Adults[a]

Antihistamine	Dosage[b]
ALKYLAMINES	
Chlorpheniramine maleate (Chlor-Trimeton, Chlorspan-12, Phenetron, Telachlor, Teldrin, Aller-Chlor, Trymegen)	4 mg q 4 to 6 hr, or 8 to 12 mg q 8 to 12 hr (SR)
Dexchlorpheniramine maleate (Polaramine, Dexchlor)	2 mg q 4 to 6 hr, or 4 to 6 mg bid (SR)
Brompheniramine maleate (Dimetane, Veltane, Bromphen, Codimal-A, Conjec B, Dehist)	4 mg q 4 to 6 hr, or 8 to 12 mg q 8 to 12 hr (SR)
Triprolidine HCl (Actidil, Myidil)	2.5 mg q 4 to 6 hr
ETHANOLAMINES	
Diphenhydramine HCl[c] (Benadryl, Benaphen, Fenylhist, Nordryl, AllerMax, Belix, Valdrene, Dormarex 2)	25 to 50 mg q 4 to 6 hr
Carbinoxamine maleate[c] (Clistin)	4 to 8 mg q 6 to 8 hr
Clemastine fumarate[c] (Tavist, Tavist-1)	1.34 to 2.68 mg q 8 to 12 hr
ETHYLENEDIAMINES	
Tripelennamine HCl (Pelamine, PBZ)	25 to 50 mg q 4 to 6 hr, or 100 mg q 12 hr (SR)
Pyrilamine maleate	25 to 50 mg q 6 to 8 hr
PHENOTHIAZINES	
Promethazine HCl[c] (Phenergan, Phenameth, Anergan, Prothazine, K-Phen, Mallergan)	12.5 to 25 mg q 6 to 24 hr
Trimeprazine[c] (Temaril)	2.5 mg q 6 hr
Methdilazine HCl[c] (Tacaryl)	8 mg q 6 to 12 hr

[a]All antihistamines listed have anticholinergic activity. All antihistamines listed have sedative effects except phenindamine.

[b]Usual adult oral dose. SR, sustained released tablets.

[c]Antiemetic effects.

Table 7.3.—*Continued*

Antihistamine	Dosage[b]
PIPERIDINES	
Cyproheptadine HCl (Periactin)	4 mg q 8 hr
Azatadine maleate (Optimine)	1 to 2 mg q 12 hr
Diphenylpyraline HCl (Hispril Spansules)	5 mg q 12 hr
Phenindamine tartrate (Nolahist)	25 mg q 4 to 6 hr
MISCELLANEOUS	
Terfenadine (Seldane)	60 mg q 12 hr

Table 7.4.
Pediatric Antihistamines

Antihistamine	Dosage
Diphenhydramine HCl	
Benadryl	>10 kg: 12.5 to 25 mg q 4 to 6 hr or 5 mg/kg/day
Benaphen	
Carbinoxamine maleate	
Clistin	>6 yr: 4 to 6 mg tid, qid 3–6 yr: 2 to 4 mg tid, qid 1–3 yr: 2 mg tid, qid
Chlorpheniramine maleate	
Chlo-Amine	6–12 yr: 2 mg q 4 to 6 hr 2–5 yr: 1 mg q 4 to 6 hr
Methdilazine HCl	
Tacaryl	>3 yr: 4 mg bid, qid
Cyproheptadine HCl	
Periactin	7–14 yr: 4 mg bid, tid 2–6 yr: 2 mg bid, tid

ANTITUSSIVES

MECHANISM OF ACTION AND INDICATIONS FOR USE:

The cough is a protective action by which irritants (dust, liquids, foreign material, etc.) and secretions are cleared from the respiratory tract. Complete cough suppression is detrimental and should be avoided. However, when the cough is disturbing, nonproductive, or potentially exhausting, agents such as antitussives are indicated. They are frequently used to relieve chronic irritation of the airways, either from the common cold or other acute upper airway infections. As with expectorants, antitussives are purely symptomatic medications that relieve the cough, but treating the *cause of the cough* should be given first priority.

Two classes of antitussives are available: narcotic (primarily codeine) and nonnarcotic. Both classes are generally central acting, suppressing the cough reflex located at the medullary cough center. There are a few nonnarcotic antitussives that act to suppress the cough reflex at its source—the stretch receptors in the respiratory passages (lungs and pleura).

CONTRAINDICATIONS:

Hypersensitivity to any component. Use with *extreme* caution in patients with chronic obstructive pulmonary disease or cor pulmonale, in patients having an acute asthmatic attack, and in patients with decreased respiratory reserve.

PRECAUTIONS:

1. The narcotic antitussives are effective cough suppressants at doses below those necessary to achieve analgesia; however, they may still exhibit respiratory depressant effects (see Chapter 16).
2. Use with caution when giving to pregnant women—these agents may cross the placental barrier.
3. Use with caution in head injury patients and patients with increased intracranial pressure—narcotic antitussives have the capacity to elevate cerebrospinal fluid pressure.
4. Antitussives are not indicated for chronic cough due to smoking, asthma, or emphysema, or where there is excessive secretion present.
5. Medical supervision is highly recommended when using these agents for patients with persistent headache, high fever, rash, nausea, or vomiting.
6. Avoid alcohol use (additive depressant effects) when taking narcotic antitussives.
7. May affect alertness; use with caution when driving or operating machinery.
8. May be addictive; use for only short periods of time.

ADVERSE REACTIONS:

Narcotic antitussives: Minimal side effects are noted when taking the usual oral dose, the most common being nausea, vomiting, sedation, dizziness, and constipation.

Nonnarcotic antitussives: Sedation, headache, dizziness, constipation, nausea, nasal congestion, hypersensitivity, GI upset.

OVERDOSAGE:

Narcotic antitussives: CNS depression, respiratory depression, respiratory or cardiac arrest (noted with rapid IV administration). 0.5 to 1 g is the lethal oral dose for codeine.

Nonnarcotic antitussives: CNS stimulation (restlessness, tremors), clonic convulsions, followed by CNS depression.

Table 7.5 lists the antitussives.

EXPECTORANTS

MECHANISM OF ACTION AND INDICATIONS FOR USE:

Expectorants increase the amount of fluid in the respiratory tract, resulting in nonproductive coughs becoming productive. Their mode of action is not clearly understood; however, some expectorants stimulate the vagal pathway innervating bronchial mucus glands. An increase in the production of bronchial secretions is induced, thereby liquefying secretions and promoting ciliary activity, making the cough less frequent. The efficacy of many of these agents is not well documented due to a lack of convincing studies.

Expectorants are used for the relief of dry, nonproductive coughs and when mucus is present in the respiratory tract. These agents are also used in the treatment of COPD, where tenacious secretions may complicate the condition.

CONTRAINDICATIONS:

Hypersensitivity to any component. Potassium iodide is contraindicated in patients with acute bronchitis, hyperthyroidism, Addison's disease, renal disease (acute or chronic), acute dehydration, and tuberculosis.

PRECAUTIONS:

1. These agents should not be used in patients with chronic or persistent coughs without first documenting the underlying condition causing the cough.
2. The best pharmacologic agent for persistent, nonproductive coughs is

Table 7.5.
Antitussives[a]

Antitussive	Dosage
Codeine	10 to 20 mg q 4 to 6 hr[b]
Dextromethorphan HBr (Mediquell, Benylin DM, Delsym, Pedia Care I, Pertussin, Congespirin, Formula 44 Cough Control Discs (with benzocaine), Sucrets Cough Control, Hold)	10 to 30 mg q 4 to 8 hr[b]
Diphenhydramine HCl (Beldin, Benylin Cough, Bydramine, Nordryl Cough, Tusstat, Valdrene, Diphen Cough)	25 mg q 4 hr[b]
Benzonatate (Tessalon Perles)	100 mg tid[b]
PEDIATRIC ANTITUSSIVES	
Codeine	6–12 yr: 5 to 10 mg q 4 to 6 hr 2–6 yr: 2.5 to 5 mg q 4 to 6 hr
Dextromethorphan HBr	
Sucrets Cough Control	6–12 yr: 5 to 10 mg q 4 hr
St. Joseph Cough Congespirin for Children	2–6 yr: 2.5 to 7.5 mg q 4 to 8 hr
PediaCare I	
Benylin DM	

[a]For a further list of narcotics that have antitussive effects, refer to Chapter 16.
[b]Usual adult oral dose.

water. Patients should increase their daily intake of fluids and breathe humidified air. Expectorants, to be effective, should be taken with a full glass of water.

ADVERSE REACTIONS:

Most common: GI upset, nausea, drowsiness.

OVERDOSAGE:

Not usually a problem; however, intensification of the effects listed under Adverse Reactions is noted.

Table 7.6 lists the expectorants.

Table 7.6.
Expectorants

Expectorant	Dosage
ADULT EXPECTORANTS	
Guaifenesin (Glycotuss, Hytuss, Gee-Gee, Breonesin, Amonidrin, Glyate, Halotussin, Malotuss, Nortussin, Robafen, Robitussin, Scot-tussin, Humibid LA, GG-Cen (syrup, 10% alcohol), Cremacoat 2 (10% alcohol), Naldecon Senior EX (alcohol free).	100 to 400 mg q 3 to 6 hr[a]
Iodine products (Potassium Iodide, SSKI, Pima, Iodo-Niacin, Hydriodic Acid)	Initially, 300 to 1000 mg after meals, tid. Then, if tolerated, 1 to 1.5 g tid.[a]
Iodinated glycerol (Iophen, R-Gen [21.75% alcohol], Organidin [elixir 21.75% alcohol])	60 mg qid[a]
Terpin Hydrate (contains 42% alcohol)	85 mg q 3 to 4 hr[a]
Miscellaneous expectorants	
Cherralex Plain	5 to 15 ml q 2 to 4 hr[a]
Ipsatol	5 to 10 ml q 3 to 4 hr[a]
PEDIATRIC EXPECTORANTS	
Guaifenesin	
Robitussin	6–12 yr: 100 to 200 mg q 3 to 6 hr
Scot-tussin	
Anti-tuss	2–6 yr: 50 to 100 mg q 4 hr
Robafen	
Miscellaneous expectorants	
Cherralex Plain	>1 yr: 2.5 to 5 ml q 4 hr
Ipsatol	3–6 yr: 5 ml q 3 to 4 hr 1–3 yr: 2.5 ml q 3 to 4 hr <1 yr: 1.25 ml q 3 to 4 hr
Rasp Cough	3–10 yr: 5 ml q 3 hr 1–3 yr: 2.5 ml q 3 hr infants: 5 to 10 drops q 3 hr

[a]Usual adult oral dose.

Table 7.7.
Cough and Cold Combinations

Trade Name	Dosage
ADULT COUGH AND COLD COMBINATIONS	
Comtrex Caplets (decongestant + antihistamine + antitussive + acetaminophen)	2 capsules q 4 hr[a]
Triaminicol Multi-Symptom Cold Tablets (decongestant + antihistamine + antitussive)	2 tablets q 4 hr[a]
CoTylenol Cold Tablets (decongestant + antihistamine + antitussive + acetaminophen)	2 tablets q 6 hr[a]
Formula 44 Cough Mixture (antihistamine + antitussive, 10% alcohol)	10 ml q 6 hr[a]
Contac Severe Cold Formula (decongestant + antihistamine + antitussive + acetaminophen, 25% alcohol)	30 ml q 6 hr or 30 ml hs[a]
NyQuil Nighttime Cold Medicine (decongestant + antihistamine + antitussive + acetaminophen, 25% alcohol)	30 ml q 6 hr or 30 ml hs[a]
Robitussin Night Relief Colds Formula Liquid (decongestant + antihistamine + antitussive + acetaminophen, 25% alcohol, saccharin, sorbitol)	30 ml hs[a]
Robitussin-PE Syrup (decongestant + expectorant)	10 ml q 4 hr[a]
Robitussin-DM Syrup (antitussive + expectorant)	10 ml q 6 to 8 hr
Robitussin-CF Syrup (decongestant + antitussive + expectorant)	10 ml q 4 hr
Sudafed Cough Syrup (decongestant + antitussive + expectorant)	20 ml q 4 to 6 hr
Formula 44M Liquid (decongestant + antitussive + expectorant)	20 ml q 6 hr
Sine-Aid Extra Strength Caplets (decongestant + acetaminophen)	2 caplets q 4 to 6 hr
Tylenol Maximum Strength Sinus Tablets and Caplets (decongestant + acetaminophen)	2 tablets q 4 to 6 hr
Coricidin Tablets (antihistamine + acetaminophen)	2 tablets q 4 hr
Chlor-Trimeton Decongestant Repetabs (decongestant + antihistamine)	1 tablet q 12 hr[a]
Allerest 12 Hour Capsules (decongestant + antihistamine)	1 capsule q 12 hr[a]
Contac 12 Hour Capsules (decongestant + antihistamine)	1 capsule q 12 hr[a]

[a]Usual adult oral dose.

Table 7.7—*Continued*

Expectorant	Dosage
Dimetapp Extentabs (decongestant + antihistamine)	1 tablet q 12 hr[a]
Sudafed Plus Tablets (decongestant + antihistamine)	1 tablet q 4 to 6 hr[a]
Triaminic Allergy Tablets (decongestant + antihistamine)	1 tablet q 4 hr[a]
PEDIATRIC COUGH AND COLD PREPARATIONS	
Naldecon-DX Pediatric Syrup (decongestant + antitussive + expectorant, 5% alcohol)	5 to 10 ml qid
Dorcol Children's Cough Syrup (decongestant + antitussive + expectorant)	5 to 10 ml q 4 hr
Bayer Cough Syrup for Children (decongestant + antitussive, 5% alcohol)	5 to 20 ml q 4 hr
Pedia Care 3 Children's Relief (decongestant + antihistamine + antitussive)	10 to 15 ml q 4 to 6 hr
Contac Jr. Liquid (decongestant + antitussive + acetaminophen)	1 dose q 4 to 6 hr

COUGH AND COLD COMBINATIONS

Table 7.7 lists some of the more commonly used and recognized over-the-counter cough and cold preparations. Refer to package brochures for specific types and amounts of decongestant, antihistamine, expectorant, or antitussive contained within the formula.

8 SYMPATHOMIMETIC BRONCHODILATORS

MECHANISM OF ACTION AND INDICATIONS FOR USE:

Sympathomimetic bronchodilators produce vasodilation and bronchodilation, inhibit histamine release from mast cells, and enhance ciliary motility. The primary determinant for use is the relative selectivity of action (i.e., β_2 stimulation) with minimal side effects. (Review Mechanism of Action within the Autonomic Nervous System in Chapter 2). These agents are indicated for the relief of acute or chronic reversible bronchospasm in asthma, bronchitis, emphysema, or bronchiectasis, and in the prevention of exercise-induced bronchospasm.

Figure 8.1 compares the various nucleus modifications of the sympathomimetic bronchodilators, and Table 8.1 summarizes the pharmacologic effects of these inhaled agents.

CONTRAINDICATIONS:

Hypersensitivity to the drug. Cardiac arrhythmias associated with tachycardia.

PRECAUTIONS:

1. Excessive use of inhalants may lead to the development of paradoxical bronchospasm and increased airway resistance. Tolerance and tachyphylaxis may also occur.
2. Concomitant use with adrenergic β blockers antagonizes the effects of bronchodilators. May also cause vasoconstriction and reflex bradycardia.
3. Use cautiously in patients with cardiovascular disease, including coronary insufficiency, cardiac arrhythmias, and history of stroke and hypertension (owing to possible toxic symptoms). Also, use with caution in patients who are unusually hyperreactive to sympathomimetic agents.

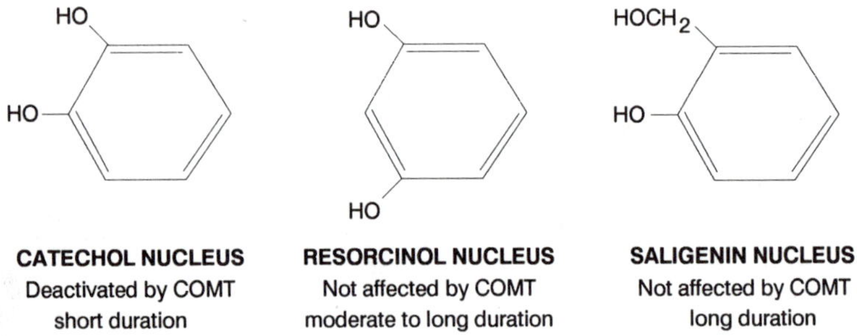

Figure 8.1. Sympathomimetic nucleus modifications.

4. If bronchial irritation, nervousness, or restlessness occurs, reduce dosage.
5. Use cautiously in pregnancy; several of these agents may cross the placental barrier.
6. Usage in children—the safety and efficacy of several of these agents in children under 12 years old have not been established.
7. Coadministered use of one sympathomimetic agent with another may produce unwanted additive effects.
8. Catecholamines must be stored in light-resistant containers. Heat, light, or air will metabolize catecholamines into inert adrenochromes.
9. Use of catecholamines with:
    a. Digitalis may produce additive effects and ectopic pacemaker activity.
    b. MAO inhibitors may create a hypertensive crisis.
    c. Diuretics and antihypertensive drugs will antagonize the effects of catecholamines.
    d. Epinephrine or isoproterenol may cause serious cardiac arrhythmias (may alternate these drugs every 4 hours).
10. If a sympathomimetic crisis occurs, the effects may be counteracted by injection of an α- or β-adrenergic blocker.
11. Catecholamines are not effective when given orally owing to inactivation in the G.I. tract and liver by the sulfatase enzymes.

ADVERSE REACTIONS:

Adverse reactions are significantly reduced with aerosol administration of these agents.

CNS: Anxiety, fear, apprehension, tremors, irritability, lightheadedness, headache, flushing, pallor, sweating, insomnia.

Cardiovascular: Hypertension, hypotension, arrhythmias, palpitations. Reflex tachycardia from peripheral vasodilation and cardiac stimulation are dose-related occurrences.

Table 8.1.
Summary of the Pharmacological Effects of the Bronchodilators[a]

Drug	α[b]	β_1[b]	β_2[b]	β_2 Potency[c]	Duration[d]
Albuterol	0	±	+ + + +	5	Long
Bitolterol	0	+ +	+ + + +	5	Long
Epinephrine	+ + +	+ + + +	+ + +	5	Short
Ephedrine	+ +	+ + +	+ + +	—	Medium
Ethylnorepinephrine	+ +	+ +	+ +	—	Short
Fenoterol	0	+	+ + + +	5	Long
Isoetharine	0	+ +	+ + +	1.7	Medium
Isoproterenol	0	+ + + +	+ + + +	10	Short
Metaproterenol	0	+ +	+ +	1	Medium
Pirbuterol	0	±	+ + + +	3	Long
Racemic epinephrine	+ +	+ + +	+ +	2	Short
Terbutaline	0	±	+ + + +	2.5	Long

[a]This information is approximate only. Many factors—such as dose given, route of administration, presence of disease, other administered drugs, or tachyphylaxis—may interact to modify the relative effects of these bronchodilators. (—) represents an unknown value.
[b]+, minor effect; + +, + + +, moderate effect; + + + +, strong effect.
[c]β_2 potency relative to metaproterenol; the larger the number, the more potent the drug.
[d]Short, ½ to 2 hours; medium, 2 to 4 hours; long, 4 to 6 hours.

Pulmonary: Coughing, bronchospasm, pulmonary edema (IV use), respiratory difficulties.

GI: Nausea, vomiting, heartburn.

OVERDOSAGE:

Inhalation: Intensification of the unwanted effects listed under Adverse Reactions may occur. May produce anginal pain and hypertension. Increased blood pressure may be initially noted, then pressure may drop, possibly causing shock. Treatment consists of supportive care and discontinuance of the drug. May cautiously use β-receptor blockers, bearing in mind the possibility of airway aggravation.

Systemic: Palpitations, tachycardia, bradycardia, heart block, chest pain, hypertension, nausea, vomiting, delirium, collapse, and coma. Treatment consists of rapid intervention to reduce the incidence of morbidity and mortality. Airway, ventilation, and cardiovascular circulation (CPR) may be indicated in severe acute toxic reactions.

In the following list of sympathomimetic bronchodilators, the generic name is given first followed by brand names. Also, MDI refers to metered dose inhaler, PO refers to the oral route, SC refers to subcutaneous injection, IM refers to intramuscular injection, IV refers to intravenous injection, and NS refers to normal saline.

ALBUTEROL (SALBUTAMOL in Europe)
PROVENTIL, VENTOLIN

Structure: Member of the saligenin group.

Mode of action: Specific β_2 activity.
Minimal β_1 activity.
No α activity.

Onset of action: 2 to 10 minutes inhalation. Within 30 minutes oral.

Peak effect: 30 to 60 minutes inhalation. 1 to 2 hours oral.

Duration: Up to 6 hours inhalation. 4 to 8 hours oral.

Dosage form: ***Inhal solution:*** 0.5% (5 mg albuterol/ml)
Inhal unit dose: 0.083% in 3 ml.
MDI: 90 μg albuterol/inhalation.
PO: a. Tablets 2, 4 mg (also extended release).
b. Syrup 2 mg per 5 ml.

Dosage: Adults and children >12 years:
Inhal solution: 2.5 mg (0.5 ml) diluted with 2.5 ml NS given q 3 to 4 hr by nebulization.
Inhal unit dose: One vial per treatment by nebulization.
MDI: 2 inhalations, with 1 minute between inhalations, repeated every 4 to 6 hours and 15 minutes prior to exercise.
PO: *Tablets,* 2 to 4 mg qid. Do not exceed total daily dose of 32 mg; adjust dosage depending on response. *Syrup,* Children 2 to 6 years: starting dose 0.1 mg/kg 3 times daily. Do not exceed 4 mg, 3 times daily. Children 6 to 14 years and adults: starting dose 2 mg qid. Do not exceed 24 mg/day in divided doses.

BITOLTEROL MESYLATE
TORNALATE

Mode of action: Specific β_2 activity.
Minimal β_1 activity.
No α activity.

Onset of action: 3 to 4 minutes.
Peak effect: 60 to 90 minutes.
Duration: 5 to 8 hours.
Dosage form: MDI: 0.8% delivers 0.37 mg bitolterol/inhalation.
Dosage: Adults and children over 12 years: 2 inhalations, with 1 to 3 minutes between inhalations, followed by a third inhalation if needed, repeated every 4 to 6 hours. Do not exceed 3 inhalations every 6 hours or 2 inhalations every 4 hours. For prevention of bronchospasm: 2 inhalations every 8 hours.

Note: Bitolterol is converted to the active drug colterol in the body. Studies indicate that colterol may be a more potent β_2 drug than isoproterenol.

EPINEPHRINE HYDROCHLORIDE

TRADE NAMES:

AEROSOL PREPARATIONS: *0.16 mg epinephrine per spray:* AsthmaHaler, Bronitin Mist, Bronkaid Mist, Medihaler-Epi, Primatene Mist. *0.2 mg epinephrine per spray:* Primatene Mist, Epinephrine (Various). *0.27 mg epinephrine per spray:* Bronkaid Mist.

SOLUTION FOR NEBULIZATION: *1:100 epinephrine HCl:* Adrenalin Chloride

SOLUTION FOR INJECTION: *1:1000 solution:* Adrenalin Chloride, Epinephrine (various). *1:200 suspension:* Sus-Phrine

ADDITIONAL INDICATIONS: For the treatment of hypersensitivity reactions to drugs, sera, insect stings or other allergens. (See also Chapter 19).

Structure: Member of the catecholamine group.
Mode of action: Marked stimulation of α, β_1, β_2 receptors. Naturally synthesized by the adrenal medulla. Causes vasoconstriction, pressor effects, cardiac stimulation, bronchodilation, and decongestion (see Chapter 19 for further information).
Onset of action: 3 to 5 minutes inhalation. 6 to 15 minutes SC. IM route variable.
Peak effect: 5 to 20 minutes inhalation.
Duration: Less than 60 minutes. (Rapidly metabolized; epinephrine $\xrightarrow{\text{COMT}}$ metanephrine)
Dosage form: ***Inhal solution:*** 1% (1:100, 10 mg/ml).

MDI: 0.16, 0.2, 0.27 mg epinephrine/inhalation.
Injection: 1:1,000 solution. 1:200 suspension.

Dosage: ***Inhal solution:*** Place 8 to 15 drops into hand bulb nebulizer reservoir. Squeeze the bulb 1 to 3 times, inhale deeply. If, after 5 minutes, relief has not occurred, administer 2 to 3 additional inhalations. May repeat up to 6 times daily. OR 0.25 to 0.5 ml diluted 1:3 with NS given by nebulization.

MDI: 1 to 2 inhalations separated by an interval of 1 to 5 minutes, administered at the first symptoms of bronchospasm.

Injection: *1:1000 solution given SC or IM:* 0.3 to 0.5 ml repeated every 20 minutes to 4 hours. For infants and children: 0.01 ml/kg SC repeated every 20 minutes to 4 hours. Do not exceed 0.5 ml per pediatric dose.

1:200 suspension given SC only: 0.1 to 0.3 ml, prn, given not more often than every 6 hours. For infants and children: 0.005 ml/kg (maximum single dose for children less than 30 kg, 0.15 ml).

Note: Epinephrine is not used in patients who also receive digitalis; synergistic activity may occur, producing serious unwanted side effects.
Nursing consideration: Never inject the 1:100 solution intended for inhalation. IV injection of this concentration has caused death.

EPHEDRINE SULFATE

Mode of action: Moderate α, β_1, β_2 activity. The actions of ephedrine are similar to epinephrine but with a longer duration (ephedrine is not a catecholamine, therefore it is not inactivated by COMT). However, ephedrine is not as effective a bronchodilator as epinephrine. Ephedrine is not available for use in the inhalational route.

Onset of action: 10 to 20 minutes IM. 15 to 60 minutes PO.

Duration: 30 to 60 minutes IM, SC, IV. 3 to 5 hours PO.

Dosage form: ***PO:*** a. Capsules 25, 50 mg.
b. Syrup 11 mg/5 ml, 20 mg/5 ml.
Injection: 25 mg/ml, 50 mg/ml

Dosage: ***All routes:*** Adults: 25 to 50 mg every 3 to 4 hours (IV route given slowly). Not to exceed total daily dose of 150 mg. Children: 3 mg/kg/day divided into 4 to 6 doses.

ETHYLNOREPINEPHRINE HYDROCHLORIDE
BRONKEPHRINE

Structure:	Member of the catecholamine group.
Mode of action:	α, β_1, and β_2 activity. Especially suited for diabetic asthmatics and patients unresponsive to epinephrine or isoproterenol. Not available for use in the inhalational route, but may be used concomitantly with aerosolized bronchodilators.
Onset of action:	6 to 12 minutes.
Duration:	1 to 2 hours.
Dosage form:	***Injection:*** 2 mg/ml supplied in 1-ml ampules.
Dosage:	***IM, SC:*** Adults, 0.5 to 1 ml. Children, 0.1 to 0.5 ml (depends on age and weight).

FENOTEROL
BEROTEC

Structure:	Member of the resorcinol group.
Mode of action:	Specific β_2 activity. Minimal β_1 activity. No α activity.
Onset of action:	3 to 4 minutes.
Peak effect:	Less than 60 minutes.
Duration:	2 to 6 hours.
Dosage form:	***MDI:*** 0.16 mg/inhalation.
Dosage:	Same as bitolterol.

ISOETHARINE HYDROCHLORIDE
BRONKOMETER, BRONKOSOL

Structure:	Member of the catecholamine group.
Mode of action:	Moderate β_2 activity. Moderate β_1 activity. No α activity.
Onset of action:	Approximately 5 minutes.
Peak effect:	15 to 60 minutes.
Duration:	1.5 to 3 hours.

Dosage form: *Inhal solution:* 1%, 0.5%
Inhal unit dose: varies from 0.062% to 0.25% in 2- to 4-ml single-dose vials.
MDI: 340 μg/inhalation (0.61%).

Dosage: Adults and children >12 years:
Inhal solution: *1.0% solution:* 0.25 to 0.5 ml diluted 1:3 with NS given every 3 to 4 hours by nebulization. *0.5% solution;* 0.5 ml diluted 1:3 with NS given every 3 to 4 hours by nebulization.
Inhal unit dose: One vial per treatment by nebulization.
MDI: 1 or 2 inhalations with 1-minute interval between inhalations.

ISOPROTERENOL
ISUPREL, VAPO-ISO, MEDIHALER-ISO

Structure: Member of the catecholamine group.

Mode of action: Purest β stimulant with strong β_1 and β_2 activity. Produces pronounced stimulation of the heart, skeletal muscle vessels, and GI tract and bronchodilation. May generate a drop in PaO_2 and blood pressure through the preferential correction of a shunt (see also Chapter 20).

Onset of action: Within 2 minutes.

Peak effect: 3 to 5 minutes.

Duration: 1.5 to 2 hours. Metabolized by COMT to 3-0-methyl isoproterenol, a weak β blocker.

Dosage form: *Inhal solution:* 0.25% (1:400), 0.5% (1:200), 1% (1:100).
Inhal unit dose: 0.031%, 0.062%, (in 4 ml).
MDI: 80 μg, 131 μg/ inhalation.
Sublingual: 10-mg, 15-mg tablets
Injection: See Chapter 20.

Dosage: *Inhal solution:* 0.25 to 0.5 ml of a 1:200 solution diluted with 2 to 2.5 ml NS (concentration of 1:800 to 1:1000) given up to 5 times daily by nebulization. For acute asthma: 5 to 15 deep inhalations of a 1:200 solution or 3 to 7 deep inhalations of a 1:100 solution given by hand bulb nebulizer, may be repeated up to 5 times daily if necessary. Children: dilute with NS 0.25 ml of the 1:200 solution and give by nebulization.

Inhal unit dose: One vial per treatment.
MDI: 1 or 2 inhalations with 2- to 5-minute intervals between inhalations. May be repeated every 3 to 4 hours.
Sublingual: 10 to 20 mg tid; not to exceed total dose of 60 mg/day
Children: 5 to 10 mg; not to exceed 30 mg/day
Parenteral route: See Chapter 20.

METAPROTERENOL SULFATE
ALUPENT, METAPREL

Structure: Member of the resorcinol group.

Mode of action: Moderate β_2 activity.
Moderate β_1 activity.
No α activity.
Similar to isoproterenol, but 1/10 as strong with fewer side effects and longer duration (not metabolized by COMT).

Onset of action: 1 to 5 minutes inhalation. 15 to 30 minutes oral.

Peak effect: 5 to 30 minutes inhalation. 60 minutes oral.

Duration: 3 to 4 hours inhalation. Up to 4 hours PO.

Dosage form: ***Inhal solution:*** 5%.
Inhal unit dose: 0.6% in 2.5-ml vials.
MDI: 0.65 mg/inhalation.
PO: a. Tablets 10, 20 mg.
b. Syrup 10 mg/5 ml.

Dosage: Adults and children >12 years:
Inhal solution: 0.3 ml (range 0.2 to 0.3 ml) diluted with 2.5 ml NS given every 3 to 4 hours by nebulization. *Hand bulb nebulizer:* 10 inhalations (range 5 to 15 inhalations) given undiluted every 3 to 4 hours.
Inhal unit dose: One vial per treatment given by nebulization.
MDI: 2 to 3 inhalations every 3 to 4 hours. Do not exceed 12 inhalations per day.
PO: 20 mg every 3 to 4 hours. Children 6 to 9 years: 10 mg every 3 to 4 hours. Children 6 to 9 years: 10 mg every 3 to 4 hours. Children <6 years: 1.3 to 2.6 mg/kg/day.

Note: Adrenergic effects may be potentiated if metaproterenol is used before or after other adrenergic bronchodilators. May use aerosol metaproterenol and tablets concomitantly. Monitor for unwanted effects.

PIRBUTEROL ACETATE
MAXAIR

Structure: Member of the saligenin group.
Mode of action: Specific β_2 activity.
Minimal β_1 activity.
No α activity.
Onset of action: Within 5 minutes.
Peak effect: 30 to 60 minutes.
Duration: Up to 5 hours.
Dosage form: ***MDI:*** 0.2 mg/inhalation.
Dosage: Adults and children >12 years:
1 to 2 inhalations every 4 to 6 hours. Do not exceed total daily dose of 12 inhalations.

RACEMIC EPINEPHRINE
MICRONEFRIN, VAPONEFRIN

Structure: Stereoisomer of epinephrine.
Mode of action: Same as epinephrine, giving both α and β stimulation; however, racemic epinephrine produces one-half the physiologic effects as epinephrine. Indicated for use in laryngotracheobronchitis, stridor, and post-extubation upper airway edema.
Onset of action: 1 to 5 minutes.
Peak effect: 5 to 15 minutes.
Duration: 1 to 3 hours.
Dosage form: ***Inhal solution:*** 1.25%, 2.25% (of epinephrine base)
Dosage: Adults and children:
0.25 to 0.5 ml diluted with 3 to 5 ml NS q 1 to 2 hr prn.

TERBUTALINE SULFATE
BRETHAIRE, BRETHINE, BRICANYL

Structure: Member of the resorcinol group.
Mode of action: Specific β_2 activity.
Minimal β_1 activity.
No α activity.
Analogue of isoproterenol. Twice as potent as metaproterenol, yet produces fewer β_1 side effects. May also be used to relax uterine muscle during premature labor.
Onset of action: 5 to 15 minutes.

Peak effect: ½ to 1 hour inhalation. PO 2 to 4 hours.

Duration: 2 to 6 hours inhalation. PO 4 to 8 hours. SC 2 to 4 hours.

Dosage form: ***MDI:*** 0.2 mg/inhalation.
PO: 2.5-, 5-mg tablets.
Injection: 1 mg/ml. The subcutaneous solution is also the current source used for inhalation.

Dosage: Adults and children >12 years:
Inhal solution: 1 to 2 mg of the 0.1% solution diluted with NS given every 2 to 4 hours by nebulization. This form of terbutaline administration is not yet approved by the FDA.
MDI: 2 inhalations with at least 60 seconds between inhalations given every 4 to 6 hours.
PO: 5 mg every 6 hours. Not to exceed 15 mg/day. Children 12 to 15 years: 2.5 mg every 6 hours. Not to exceed 7.5 mg/day.
Injection: SC only; 0.25 mg. A second dose of 0.25 mg may be administered if patient does not respond to the first dose. Do not exceed a total dose of 0.5 mg in 4 hours. Consider other therapeutic agents if patient fails to respond to the second dose.

9 ANTICHOLINERGIC (ANTIMUSCARINIC) BRONCHODILATORS

ATROPINE

MECHANISM OF ACTION AND INDICATIONS FOR USE:

Atropine produces its beneficial bronchodilating effect by two mechanisms: it competitively inhibits the actions of acetylcholine at muscarinic receptors (Fig. 9.1) and it inhibits acetylcholine-enhanced mast cell degranulation. (review Mechanism of Action within the Autonomic Nervous System in Chapter 2).

Other effects of atropine include decreased salivary and bronchial secretion, increased heart rate through the suppression of parasympathetic (vagal) stimulation, relaxation of GI tone and motility, and suppression of gastric acid secretion.

Atropine is indicated for use:

1. In cholinergic-mediated bronchospasm.
2. As a supplement in peptic ulcer therapy.
3. As a preoperative drying agent to control bronchial, nasal, pharyngeal, and salivary secretions.
4. As an antidote for mushroom poisoning (*Amanita muscaria* species) and chemical warfare nerve gases.
5. As a resuscitative measure during cardiac arrest (see also Chapter 19). Also, because of atropine's vagolytic actions, it is especially suited for use in patients with hypotension associated with sinus bradycardia, junctional bradycardia, third-degree AV block, and second-degree AV block (Mobitz Types I and II).

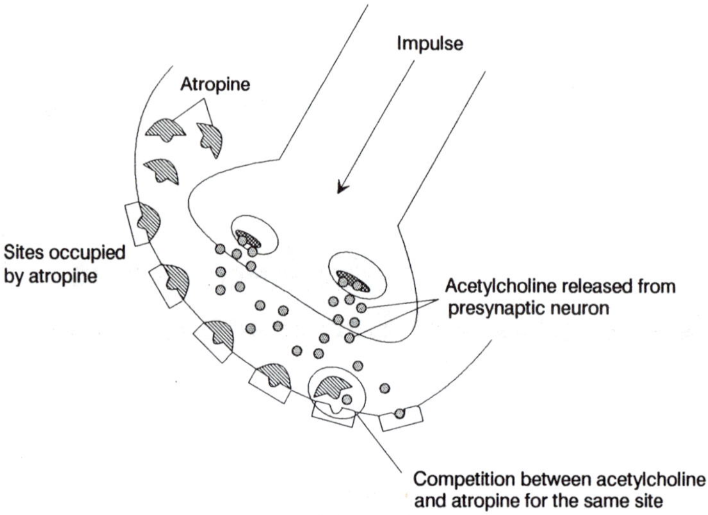

Figure 9.1. Graphic presentation of competitive inhibition by atropine. (Adapted from Teplitz L. *Nursing 89: clinical close-up on atropine.* Springhouse, PA: Springhouse Corporation, 1989.)

6. To prevent reflex bradycardia such as that induced by oropharyngeal stimulation during intubation.

CONTRAINDICATIONS:

Hypersensitivity to the drug. Glaucoma, prostatic hypertrophy, and tachycardia. Unstable cardiovascular status in acute hemorrhage, and myocardial ischemia.

PRECAUTIONS:

1. CNS stimulation may be noted with increased dosages.
2. Following inhalation, systemic absorption may occur. Nondetectable to highly significant symptoms of unwanted side effects may result.
3. Safety and efficacy of use during pregnancy and use in children have not been established.
4. Use in patients with chronic lung disease may precipitate mucus plugging.
5. Use with extreme caution in the myasthenia gravis patient. However, atropine may be given to reverse the effects of cholinergic muscle stimulants in cases of overdose (see Chapter 10).

ADVERSE REACTIONS:

CNS: Headache, nervousness, drowsiness, dizziness, insomnia, fever, confusion, agitation.

Cardiovascular: Bradycardia (low doses), tachycardia (higher doses), palpitations, angina.

Pulmonary: Thickening of secretions, mucus plugging.

GI: Dry nose and mouth, thirst, nausea, vomiting, dysphagia, heartburn.

Side effects of atropine are dose related:

Dose	Effects
0.5 mg:	Slight decrease in cardiac function, slight dryness of mouth, reduced sweating.
1.0 mg:	Increased dryness of mouth, thirst, and cardiac rate. Slight dilation of pupil.
2.0 mg:	Rapid cardiac rate, palpitations, increased dryness of mouth, dilated pupils, slight blurring of vision.
5.0 mg:	Marked unwanted side effects as mentioned above, in addition to difficulty in swallowing, restlessness, fatigue, headache, difficulty in micturition, and decreased intestinal peristalsis.
10 mg or more:	Above symptoms markedly pronounced, in addition to rapid and weak pulse, very blurred vision, hot, flushed, dry skin, ataxia, hallucinations, delirium, coma.

OVERDOSAGE:

As dosage is increased, adverse reactions are intensified, possibly leading to delirium, hallucinations, or coma. Individual tolerance varies; however, toxic effects are primarily dose related and are more commonly seen in children.

Treatment with IV physostigmine (reverses muscarinic blockade, see also Chapter 10) is reserved for patients with severe drug induced supraventricular tachycardia.

Onset of action:	Approximately 15 minutes.
Peak effect:	1 to 2 hours.
Duration:	3 to 6 hours (dose dependent).
Dosage form:	***Inhal solution:*** 0.4 mg/ml, in unit dose: 1 mg/0.5 ml (0.2%), 2.5 mg/0.5 ml (0.5%). ***PO:*** 0.4-mg tablets. ***Injection:*** Varies from 0.05 to 1.2 mg/ml.

Dosage: *Inhal solution:* Range 0.8 mg to 2.5 mg (or: adults 0.025 mg/kg, children 0.05 mg/kg) diluted with 3 to 5 ml NS given 3 to 4 times daily by nebulization. Do not exceed 2.5 mg per dose.
PO: 0.4 mg to 0.6 mg every 4 to 6 hours. Children: 0.01 mg/kg up to 0.4 mg per dose every 4 to 6 hours.
Injection: 0.5 mg per dose (range 0.4 to 0.6 mg). Children: 0.1 mg in the newborn up to 0.6 mg in a 12-year-old.
For bradyarrhythmias: 0.5 mg to 1 mg every 1 to 2 hours as needed, up to a maximum of 2 mg per dose. Children: 0.01 to 0.03 mg/kg up to a maximum of 0.4 mg per dose.

Note: When atropine is used concomitantly with sympathomimetic bronchodilators, useful additive effects are noted. This is possibly due to atropine's ability to dilate large airways to a greater extent than small airways.

IPRATROPIUM BROMIDE
ATROVENT

Mode of action: Derivative of atropine, essentially the same action as atropine, yet without the systemic side effects. Dryness of mouth may occur; however, ipratropium does not produce thickening or plugging of mucus secretions. Duovent (a combination of ipratropium bromide and fenoterol) is currently marketed in Great Britain in MDI form. Advantages to this combination include the beneficial additive effects of combining an antimuscarinic agent (upper airway bronchodilation) with a β_2 selective bronchodilator (lower airway bronchodilation).

Onset of action: 15 minutes.

Peak effect: 1 to 2 hours.

Duration: 4 to 6 hours.

Dosage form: *MDI:* 18 μg/inhalation.

Dosage: Adults and children over 12 years: 1 to 2 inhalations qid, not to exceed 12 inhalations in 24 hours.

Note: Temporary blurring of vision may occur if sprayed into eyes. Ipratropium is not well absorbed systemically, therefore overdosage by inhalation is not likely.

GLYCOPYRROLATE
ROBINUL

Glycopyrrolate is a new experimental aerosol antimuscarinic bronchodilator. This quaternary ammonium derivative of atropine has the same indications and uses as atropine, yet produces fewer CNS side effects than atropine. Glycopyrrolate is supplied as an injection solution of 0.2 mg/ml. For aerosol administration a 1-mg dose diluted with NS is given tid or qid. Onset of action is noted within 30 minutes, with a peak effect in 1 to 2 hours. Glycopyrrolate has a relatively long duration of activity of 6 to 8 hours.

OXITROPIUM BROMIDE
Ba 235

A derivative of scopolamine, oxitropium bromide is currently under investigation as an aerosol antimuscarinic bronchodilator. Supplied in MDI form, a 200-μg dose elicits a peak effect within 1 to 2 hours with a long-duration of activity of 6 to 8 hours.

10
Cholinergic Muscle Stimulants

MECHANISM OF ACTION AND INDICATIONS FOR USE:

Cholinergic agents increase acetylcholine's duration of action at the cholinergic nicotinic receptor site by inhibiting the hydrolysis of acetylcholine by the enzyme acetylcholinesterase (Fig. 10.1). By this action, the transmission of impulses are facilitated at the myoneural junction, enhancing muscular strength and response to repetitive nerve stimulation.

Cholinergic agents are indicated for use in the diagnosis and treatment of myasthenia gravis and for reversal of nondepolarizing muscle relaxants.

CONTRAINDICATIONS:

Hypersensitivity to these drugs, intestinal and urinary obstructions.

PRECAUTIONS:

1. Use with extreme caution in patients with asthma, epilepsy, bradycardia, recent coronary occlusion, hyperthyroidism, cardiac arrhythmias, or peptic ulcer owing to the possible aggravation of symptoms or increase in the severity of these diseases with cholinergic agonist use.
2. Anticholinesterase insensitivity may occur with repeated use of these drugs. Reduce or withhold dosage until the patient again becomes sensitive. Monitor patient for myasthenic crisis.
3. Have atropine sulfate readily available for possible overdose of these agents or when large doses are given, prior injection of atropine sulfate is recommended.

ADVERSE REACTIONS:

CNS: Convulsions, dysphonia, dizziness, drowsiness, loss of consciousness, headache.

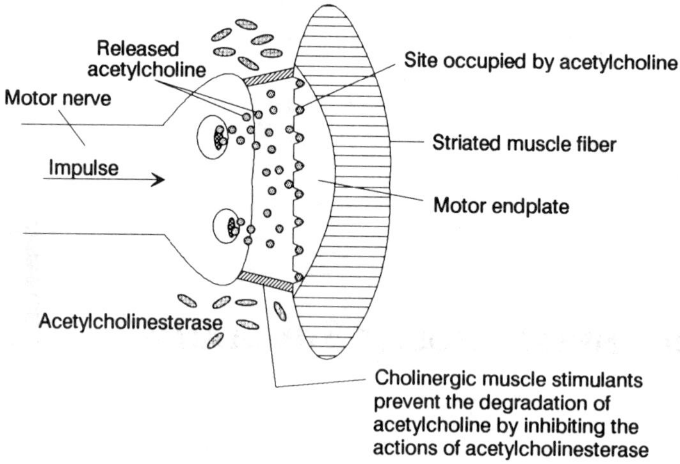

Figure 10.1. The actions of cholinergic muscle stimulants at the myoneural junction.

Cardiovascular: Bradycardia, tachycardia, other arrhythmias, decreased cardiac output, hypotension, cardiac arrest, syncope.

Pulmonary: Increased tracheobronchial secretions, laryngospasm, bronchoconstriction, dyspnea, respiratory depression, respiratory arrest.

GI: Increased salivary, gastric, and intestinal secretions, nausea, vomiting, dysphagia, increased peristalsis, diarrhea, abdominal cramps.

Miscellaneous: Urinary frequency and urgency, diaphoresis, rash, flushing.

OVERDOSAGE:

Marked pronouncement of parasympathomimetic actions; cardiac arrhythmias, increased GI stimulation, abdominal cramps, diarrhea, vomiting, excessive salivation, blurring of vision, paralysis of voluntary muscles. Also, conversion of a myasthenia crisis to a cholinergic crisis has been noted with excessive use of anticholinesterase drugs.

Treatment consists of discontinuing all cholinergic medications and administering from 0.5 to 1.0 mg of atropine IV. A total dose of 5 to 10 mg of atropine may be required. Monitor patient for supportive treatment such as assisted respirations, intubation, oxygen, etc.

AMBENONIUM CHLORIDE
MYTELASE

Indications: Administered orally to treat myasthenia gravis. Ambenonium has a longer duration of action than other anticholinesterase agents, therefore requircs less frequency of use. It produces less side effects and is the preferred drug in patients who are allergic to the bromide ion found in other cholinergic muscle stimulants.

Onset of action: 20 to 30 minutes.

Duration: 3 to 8 hours.

Dosage form: ***PO:*** 10-mg tablets.

Dosage: *Adults:*

5 to 25 mg 3 to 4 times daily. Start with 5 mg and increase gradually to determine optimal dose. Dosage must be adjusted at 1- to 2-day intervals to avoid accumulation and overdosage.

Children: 0.3 mg/kg daily in divided doses, up to 1.5 mg/kg daily.

EDROPHONIUM CHLORIDE
TENSILON, ENLON

Indication: Used in the diagnosis of myasthenia gravis; however, because of its short duration, edrophonium is not useful in the maintenance or continued treatment of myasthenic patients. This drug is also used as a nondepolarizing muscle relaxant antagonist.

Onset of action: < 1 minute IV. 2 to 10 minutes IM.

Duration: 0.08 to 0.33 hours IV. 0.17 to 0.67 hours IM.

Dosage form: ***IV, IM solution:*** 10 mg/ml.

Dosage: *Adults:*

For diagnosis: Inject 2 mg IV in 15 to 30 seconds; if no reaction occurs, inject 8 mg more. Test may be repeated after 1 to 2 hours. Myasthenic patients will show an increase in muscle strength in 1 to 3 minutes which lasts for 5 to 10 minutes. Atropine should be readily available if needed.

Children:

For diagnosis: <34 kg, inject 1 mg. >34 kg, inject 2 mg. If no response occurs an additional dose of up to 5 mg in children <34 kg, and up to 10 mg in children >34 kg should be given.

For differential diagnosis of myasthenic crisis vs cholinergic crisis: Adults: inject 1 to 2 mg; if the crisis is myasthenic, the test will clearly improve respirations in the patient. If the crisis is cholinergic (indicating an overdose of medication), edrophonium will increase secretions and further weaken respiratory muscles. Only initiate this test if assisted ventilation and intubation are immediately available.

NEOSTIGMINE
PROSTIGMIN

Indication: For control and treatment of myasthenia gravis. Corticosteroids may be used as an adjunct in severe cases. Neostigmine is also used as an antidote for nondepolarizing neuromuscular blocking agents.

Onset of action: 4 to 8 minutes IV. 20 to 30 minutes IM. 45 to 75 minutes PO.

Duration: 2 to 4 hours IV, IM, PO.

Dosage form: ***IV, IM, SC solution:*** 0.25 mg/ml in 1 ml vials; 0.5 mg/ml in 1 and 10 ml vials; 1 mg/ml in 10 ml vials.
PO: 15 mg tablets.

Dosage: *Adults:*
IM, SC: 0.5 mg, adjust dosage according to patient response.
IV: 1 mg in 100 ml of saline infused at 25 ml/hr.
PO: Varies from 15 to 375 mg/day according to the response of the patient. Average dose is 150 mg in a 24 hour period.
Children:
IV, IM, SC: 0.01 to 0.04 mg/kg q 2 to 3 hour as needed.
PO: 2 mg/kg daily in divided doses.

PYRIDOSTIGMINE BROMIDE
MESTINON, REGONOL

Indication: Given orally, pyridostigmine is the most widely used cholinergic muscle stimulant for the treatment of myasthenia gravis. Individualized doses are necessary because of the wide variance in the drug's absorption, biotransformation, and elimination among patients. Pyridostigmine is also used to reverse nondepolarizing muscle relaxant effects.

Onset of action: 2 to 5 minutes IV, <15 minutes IM. 20 to 30 minutes PO.

Duration: 2 to 4 hours IV, IM. 3 to 6 hours PO.

Dosage form: ***IV, IM solution:*** 5 mg/ml.

PO: 60-mg tablets; 180-mg sustained release tablets; 60 mg/5 ml syrup.

Dosage: *Adults:*

IV, IM: Given when oral therapy is not practicable or for exacerbation; 1/30th of the oral dose, either IM or very slowly IV.

PO: Must be individualized; Initial dose of 60 to 120 mg q 3 to 4 hours.

Children:

IV, IM: For newborn infants of myasthenic mothers; 0.05 to 0.15 mg/kg.

PO: 7 mg/kg daily in divided doses (5 to 6 doses).

PHYSOSTIGMINE SALICYLATE
ANTILIRIUM

Indication: As an antidote to reverse toxic CNS effects produced by anticholinergic drugs. Physostigmine may also counteract the CNS depressant effects of diazepam. Unlabeled use includes treatment of Alzheimer's disease.

Onset of action: Peak effects are noted within 5 minutes.

Duration: Approximately 1 hour.

Dosage form: ***IM, IV:*** 1 mg/ml.

Dosage: *Adults:*

For overdosage of anticholinergics: 2 mg.

Children:

For life-threatening occurrences only: 0.02 mg/kg.

Neuromuscular Blocking Agents 11

Neuromuscular blocking agents affect the somatic motoneurons of the peripheral nervous system. This system innervates striated muscle fibers such as the biceps, triceps, deltoids, and diaphragm (i.e., body movements, posture, lifting, and breathing functions). The action of these skeletal muscles are both movements under conscious voluntary control and reflex movements, as opposed to the involuntary movements of the smooth muscle cells innervated by the autonomic nervous system.

Review of Skeletal Muscle Contraction

A motor neuron originates from the spinal cord and extends to the muscle it innervates, where it then branches into several muscle fibers. Upon stimulation, the nerve fibers shorten as a unit and the muscle contracts. Flaccidity is the relaxed state of the muscle when there is no impulse transmission occurring. The neuromuscular junction (Fig. 11.1) is the area between the motor nerve fiber and the skeletal muscle fiber. The motor endplate is the chemical receptor area for the neurotransmitter acetylcholine. When the motor endplate is chemically stimulated by acetylcholine (acetylcholine is then rapidly degraded by cholinesterase), a transient change in the membrane permeability is brought about that allows the influx of sodium ions. The influx of sodium ions across the nerve fiber membrane reverses the polarity of the muscle fiber, causing depolarization to occur. Once in the depolarized mode, the muscle fiber releases calcium. The release of calcium then initiates muscle contraction. As long as calcium is allowed to remain free, the muscle contraction continues. As depolarization ceases, calcium is taken back into its

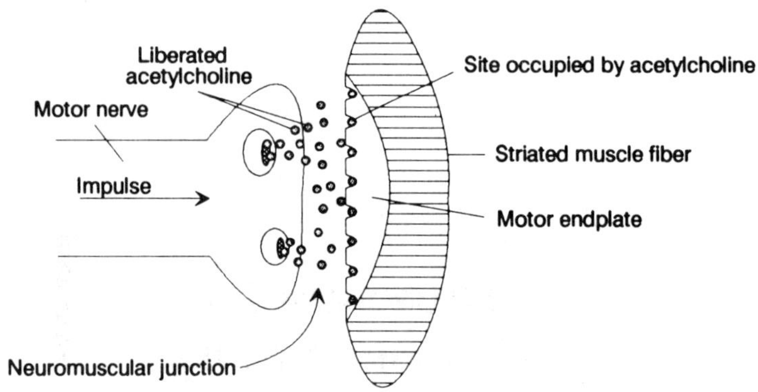

Figure 11.1. Impulse transmission across the neuromuscular junction.

storage sacs in the muscle fiber; contraction of the muscle ceases, repolarization occurs, and the membrane returns to its resting level. The entire event of muscle stimulation, depolarization, and repolarization occurs in approximately 20 milliseconds (Fig. 11.2).

MECHANISM OF ACTION AND INDICATIONS FOR USE:

Neuromuscular blocking agents prevent acetylcholine stimulation at the motor endplate by combining with and occupying these specific receptors (Fig. 11.3). By inhibiting these receptors to acetylcholine stimulation, neuromuscular blocking agents prevent muscle contraction and induce temporary muscle immobility (paralysis).

Neuromuscular blocking agents consist of two classes: nondepolarizing agents and depolarizing agents. Nondepolarizing agents competitively engage the receptor site in the muscle cell, blocking the action of acetylcholine. Nondepolarizing agents are also called curariform because their mode of action resembles the poison curare. Depolarizing agents initially instigate muscle contraction (mimicking acetylcholine), then sustain depolarization time (receptors cannot respond to acetylcholine while in a depolarized mode). Any further stimulation to the muscle is prevented until the depolarizing agent's effect is terminated. Only when the effect wears off or is hydrolyzed by pseudocholinesterase is the depolarized receptor allowed to return to its normal state of activities.

Neuromuscular blocking agents are indicated for use as an adjunct to anesthesia to induce skeletal muscle relaxation during surgery, during endotracheal intubation, and as an aid in the prevention of laryngospasm. These agents are also used as an aid to electroshock therapy to prevent fractures and to reduce the severity of convulsions, as an aid to decrease muscle spasms during seizures and

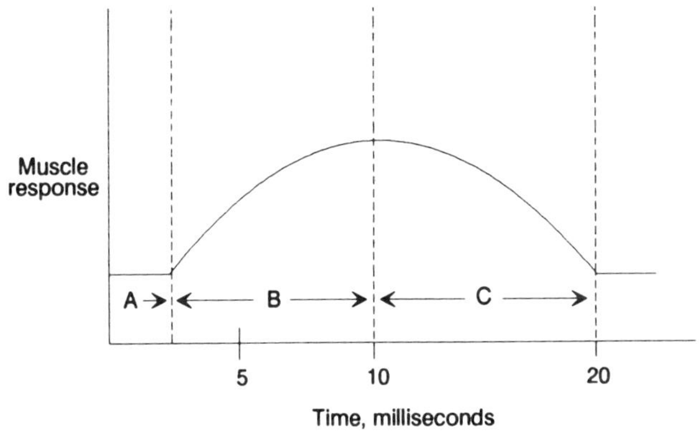

Figure 11.2. Skeletal muscle contraction. *A,* latent period; *B,* contraction; *C,* relaxation.

tetanus, and as an aid to diagnose myasthenia gravis (Only tubocurarine and when the results of tests with cholinergic muscle stimulants prove inconclusive). Nondepolarizing agents are also indicated for use to facilitate prolonged mechanical ventilation among patients who otherwise would be difficult to ventilate.

CONTRAINDICATIONS:

Hypersensitivity to these drugs. Each agent has specific contraindications to its use; therefore, additional contraindications are listed with each drug.

PRECAUTIONS:

1. Respiratory depression and apnea may follow the use of these drugs. Endotracheal intubation with assisted respirations should be immediately available.
2. These drugs have no effect on pain threshold or consciousness. Use only with adequate anesthesia.
3. Use with caution in patients with myasthenia gravis and in patients with cardiovascular, renal, hepatic, pulmonary, or endocrine dysfunction owing to prolonged muscle weakness and hypotension.
4. Use with extreme caution in patients in which histamine release is a known hazard.
5. Have antidotes readily available (neostigmine, edrophonium, pyridostigmine).

ADVERSE REACTIONS:

Most Frequent: Sustained pharmacologic action of the drug.

Cardiovascular: Bradycardia, tachycardia, blood pressure changes, cardiac arrest, arrhythmias.

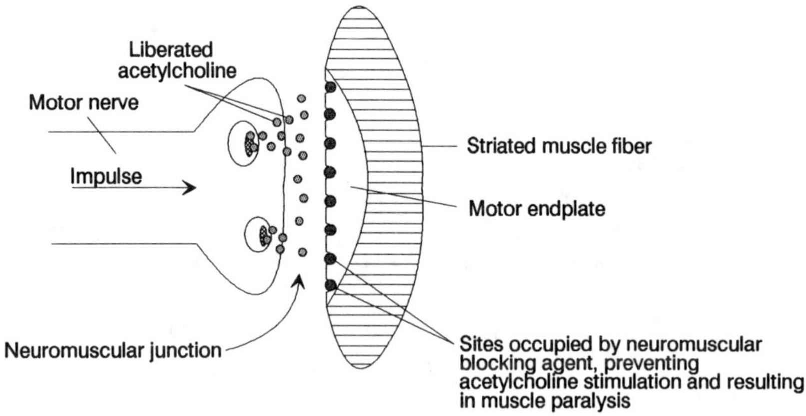

Figure 11.3. Competitive inhibition by nondepolarizing neuromuscular blocking agents.

Pulmonary: Respiratory depression, apnea, bronchoconstriction (with histamine release).
GI: Excessive salivation.
Refer to each drug for specific adverse reactions.

OVERDOSAGE:

Sustained apnea, cardiovascular collapse, prolonged muscle weakness, release of histamine. Treatment consists of ventilatory support and the administration of a cholinergic muscle stimulant such as neostigmine, pyridostigmine, or edrophonium (only effective for antagonizing the effects of nondepolarizing blocking agents).

NONDEPOLARIZING NEUROMUSCULAR BLOCKING AGENTS

ATRACURIUM BESYLATE
TRACRIUM

Mode of action: Nondepolarizing neuromuscular blocking agent that competitively engages the neuromuscular receptor site, antagonizing the effects of acetylcholine at the motor endplate. May cause the release of histamine.

Onset of action: Maximum neuromuscular blockage is achieved within 3 to 5 minutes after injection.

Duration: 20 to 40 minutes.

Dosage form: ***IV solution:*** 10 mg/ml in 5- and 10-ml vials.

Dosage: *Adults:*
0.4 to 0.5 mg/kg initial dose. Maintenance dose, 0.08 to 0.1 mg/kg given approximately q 30 min.
Children:
2 years old and above; same as adult dose. Children <2 years old; 0.3 to 0.4 mg/kg.

Adverse reactions: Histamine release symptoms; hypotension, erythema, tachycardia, circulatory collapse, edema, bronchospasm.

Contraindications: Patients with myasthenia gravis, electrolyte disorders, bronchial asthma.

GALLAMINE TRIETHIODIDE
FLAXEDIL

Mode of action: Nondepolarizing blocking agent that does not cause the release of histamine or produce bronchospasm.

Onset of action: Immediate.

Duration: 20 minutes.

Dosage form: ***IV solution:*** 100 mg/ml in 1-ml vials. 20 mg/ml in 10-ml vials.

Dosage: *Adults:*
Individualized: initial 1 mg/kg up to 100 mg. Maintenance dose: 0.5 to 1.0 mg/kg approximately q 30 minutes.
Children:
Infants up to 1 month: initially 1 mg/kg. Maintenance dose: 0.5 mg/kg.

Adverse reactions: Sinus tachycardia (blocks the cardiac vagus), hypertension, increased cardiac output, anaphylaxis.

Contraindications: Hypersensitivity to iodide, myasthenia gravis, patients at risk of increased heart rate, impaired renal function, shock.

Note: A precipitate will form if gallamine is mixed with anesthetic gases. Do not administer solution with a visible precipitate.

The presence of respiratory acidosis diminishes the blocking effects of gallamine, and alkalosis enhances the blocking action of gallamine.

METOCURINE IODIDE
METUBINE

Mode of action: Nondepolarizing blocking agent that may cause the release of histamine. Metocurine is twice as potent, yet produces fewer circulatory system effects as tubocurarine.

Onset of action: Within 2 minutes.

Duration: 25 to 90 minutes.

Dosage form: ***IV Solution:*** 2 mg/ml in 20-ml vials.

Dosage: *Adults:* Initially 0.2 to 0.4 mg/kg for endotracheal intubation. Supplemental doses average 0.5 to 1 mg. For electroshock therapy: 1.75 to 5.5 mg (average dose 2 to 3 mg).

Adverse reactions: Allergic reactions to drug or to iodide. Histamine release symptoms; hypotension, erythema, tachycardia, circulatory collapse, edema, bronchospasm.

Contraindications: Patients sensitive to iodide.

Note: When used with succinylcholine, an additive effect is noted. Do not mix metocurine with alkaline solutions (barbiturates), for a precipitate may occur.

PANCURONIUM BROMIDE
PAVULON

Mode of action: Nondepolarizing blocking agent that is similar to tubocurarine; however, pancuronium is 5 times as potent and rarely causes histamine release and does not cause hypotension due to ganglionic blocking action. Pancuronium is the drug of choice to facilitate endotracheal intubation and mechanical ventilation.

Onset of action: $<$1 minute.

Duration: 60 minutes.

Dosage form: ***IV solution:*** 1 mg/ml in 10-ml vials. 2 mg/ml in 2- and 5-ml vials, syringes.

Dosage: *Adults and children:*
Initially, 0.04 to 0.1 mg/kg.
For endotracheal intubation: 0.1 mg/kg IV bolus. (Maximum neuromuscular blocking action occurs within 2 minutes).

Adverse reactions: Salivation, skin rash, tachycardia.

Contraindications: Hypersensitivity to bromide.

Note: Acetylcholine decreases the blocking effect of pancuronium. Concomitant use with succinylcholine increases the intensity and duration of action of pancuronium.

TUBOCURARINE (CURARE) CHLORIDE

Mode of action: Produces a nondepolarizing blockade at the neuromuscular junction. Causes paralysis of all skeletal muscles. Cumulative effects may occur. A small therapeutic index exists between the therapeutic dose and the toxic dose. Tubocurarine causes the release of histamine.

Onset of action: <2 minutes.

Duration: 25 to 90 minutes.

Dosage form: ***IV solution:*** 3 mg/ml in 10-, 20-ml vials and 5-ml syringes.

Dosage: *Adults and children:* Initially, 0.2 to 0.5 mg/kg; then 0.04 to 0.1 mg/kg.

For endotracheal intubation: 0.5 to 0.6 mg/kg.

For electroshock therapy: 1.1 units/kg (initial dose is 20 units less for safety factor).

For diagnosis of myasthenia gravis: Very small doses produce an intense exaggeration of this syndrome (usually 1/15 to 1/5 of the electroshock therapy dose). The test is usually terminated within 2 to 3 minutes with the administration of neostigmine. Precaution: carefully monitor patient.

Adverse reactions: Hypotension due to ganglionic blocking; bronchospasm and all other symptoms due to histamine release.

Contraindications: Use with extreme caution in patients with renal, liver, circulatory, or pulmonary dysfunction. Also, in patients in which histamine release is a definite hazard.

Note: Respiratory acidosis and hypokalemia enhance the neuromuscular blocking effect and respiratory alkalosis diminishes the blocking action.

VECURONIUM BROMIDE
NORCURON

Mode of action: Nondepolarizing neuromuscular agent that is similar to pancuronium although slightly more potent, and 4 times more potent than atracurium. Vecuronium does not cause the release of histamine and rarely causes heart rate changes or blood pressure changes.

Onset of action: 2.5 to 3 minutes.

Duration: 25 to 40 minutes.

Dosage form: *IV solution:* 10 mg powder in 5- and 10-ml vials with diluent.

Dosage: *Adults:*
Individualized dose: 0.08 to 0.1 mg/kg as IV bolus. Maintenance dose: 0.01 to 0.015 mg/kg 25 to 40 minutes after the initial dose. Thereafter, given in 12- to 15-minute intervals.
Children:
Not recommended in neonates. 1 to 10 years: May require a slightly higher dose and more frequent supplementation than adults 10 to 17 years: Same as adult dose.

Adverse reactions: Only as pertaining to this class of drugs, due to an extension of its pharmacological action (e.g., skeletal muscle weakness, respiratory insufficiency, apnea).

Contraindications: Hypersensitivity to bromide.

DEPOLARIZING NEUROMUSCULAR BLOCKING AGENTS

SUCCINYLCHOLINE CHLORIDE
ANECTINE, QUELICIN, SUCOSTRIN, SUX-CERT

Mode of action: Depolarizing neuromuscular blocking agent that combines with the receptors of the motor endplate. Succinylcholine's effect initially excites skeletal muscle (mimics acetylcholine); then sustains the depolarization time at these receptors, preventing acetylcholine receptor stimulation. Succinylcholine is used as an adjunct to general anesthesia during surgery and during endotracheal intubation and to reduce the severity of convulsions during electroshock therapy. Succinylcholine is not generally used to facilitate mechanical ventilation due to its very short duration of action (rapidly hydrolyzed by pseudocholinesterase).

Onset of action: 1 minute.

Duration: 4 to 6 minutes.

Recovery: 8 to 10 minutes.

Dosage form:	*IV, IM solution:* 20 mg/ml in 10-ml vials. 50 mg/ml in 10-ml amps. 100 mg/ml in 10-ml vials. 100 mg powder in 5-ml vial with diluent. 500 mg powder or 1 g/vial.
Dosage:	*Adults:* *IV:* initially 0.6 to 1 mg/kg. For continuous infusion: 0.1% (1 mg/ml) or 0.2% (2 mg/ml) given at a rate of 5 to 7.5 mg/min (range, 0.5 to 10 mg/min), or 0.1 mg/kg/min. *IM:* up to 2.5 mg/kg; not to exceed 150 mg total dose. *Children:* *IV:* 2 mg/kg for infants and younger children. 1 mg/kg for older children. *IM:* 2 to 3 mg/kg; not to exceed 150 mg per dose.
Adverse reactions:	Histamine-induced symptoms, along with bradycardia, tachycardia, blood pressure changes, cardiac arrest, arrhythmias, severe respiratory depression, apnea.
Contraindications:	Use with caution in hepatic, renal, cardiovascular, or pulmonary impairments, as the action, duration, and effect of succinylcholine may be altered. Relative contraindications include patients with severe burns, tetanus, spinal cord injuries, or multiple trauma, as severe ventricular arrhythmias or cardiac arrest may occur due to the increase in plasma potassium levels following depolarization of the sensitized denervated muscle.

Note: The effects of succinylcholine may be potentiated with the administration of anticholinesterase drugs such as neostigmine or pyridostigmine, in contrast to the nondepolarizing agents, whose effects are diminished with the administration of anticholinesterase drugs.

XANTHINE BRONCHODILATORS 12

Caffeine, theophylline, and theobromine compose the group known as the methylxanthines. All three agents have the same general pharmacologic effects; however, only theophylline and its derivatives are used as bronchodilators.

MECHANISM OF ACTION AND INDICATIONS FOR USE:

For many years theophylline's mechanism of bronchodilation was believed to be through phosphodiesterase inhibition. However, recent studies indicate that some forms of theophylline that have potent bronchodilator actions have little efficacy as phosphodiesterase inhibitors. Therefore, several other mechanisms have been proposed, but as yet none have been established as being responsible for theophylline's bronchodilating effect. Other proposed mechanisms of action for theophylline include:

- Interactions with prostaglandins, calcium, or cAMP protein kinase activation.
- Reduction of catecholamine uptake or metabolism.
- Adenosine receptor antagonist (activation of the adenosine receptors located in airway smooth muscle provokes bronchoconstriction and histamine release. By blocking the actions of this receptor, theophylline produces bronchodilation and inhibits mediator release from the mast cell.)

Although the mechanism of action of theophylline is not clearly understood, its various pharmacologic effects are well known. Not only is theophylline a potent bronchodilator, but it is also a pulmonary vasodilator, a central respiratory stimulant, and a CNS stimulant. Theophylline also produces diuretic actions, inhibits uterine contractions, increases gastric acid secretion, generates positive chronotropic and inotropic effects, stimulates diaphragmatic contractility, and enhances the synthesis and release of norepinephrine and epinephrine by the adrenal medulla.

Theophylline is indicated for use in acute and chronic reversible bronchospasm, in the treatment of acute pulmonary edema (it decreases peripheral vascular resistance and venous pressure), in relieving paroxysmal nocturnal dyspnea due to left ventricular failure, and as an adjunct in the treatment of neonatal apnea and bradycardia (it produces CNS stimulation at the medullary level).

CONTRAINDICATIONS:

Hypersensitivity to the drug or any of its ingredients. May also be contraindicated in patients with active peptic ulcer, active gastritis, uncontrolled hypertension, coronary artery disease, angina pectoris, uncontrolled seizures, and uncontrolled arrhythmias.

PRECAUTIONS:

1. Ideal body weight must be used for dosage calculations. Dosage calculations must be adjusted according to the serum theophylline level.
2. Slow infusion of aminophylline (10 to 20 minutes) must be maintained. Rapid IV infusion may result in hyperventilation, hypotension, syncope, cardiac collapse, and death.
3. Use with caution in patients with severe cardiac disease, severe hypoxemia, hepatic or renal disease, severe hypertension, acute myocardial injury, cor pulmonale, and CHF and in the elderly and neonates. The volume of distribution, clearance, half-life, and excretion of these drugs may be altered in such a way as to produce toxic conditions, even with low doses.
4. The therapeutic blood level is close to the toxic level; careful monitoring of the patient is essential, including taking frequent vital signs and serum theophylline levels.
5. Concurrent use of xanthines with other xanthines or with β_2-adrenergic agonists may produce synergistic toxicity, especially in patients with compromised cardiac function, resulting in life-threatening cardiac arrhythmias.

ADVERSE REACTIONS:

Side effects are dose-related occurrences.

CNS: Headache, insomnia, dizziness, seizures, depression, irritability, restlessness, convulsions, abnormal speech, abnormal behavior.

Cardiovascular: Hypotension, arrhythmias, palpitations, tachycardia, circulatory failure.

Pulmonary: Tachypnea, respiratory arrest.

GI: Nausea, vomiting, diarrhea, anorexia, epigastric pain, hematemesis.

Miscellaneous: Fever, flushing, hyperglycemia, rash.

OVERDOSAGE:

Rapid IV infusion has caused severe cardiac arrhythmias and cardiac arrest. The first signs of toxicity may be convulsions or ventricular arrhythmias. In children, seizures and death may be the first sign of toxicity. Other toxic symptoms include a marked reaction from one or more of the effects listed under Adverse Reactions. Treatment consists of:

- Discontinuing the administration of the xanthine;
- Providing supportive care;
- Inducing vomiting (only if seizures have not occurred); and
- Guarding against the possibility of aspiration in patients with impaired consciousness, in infants, and in children.

If seizures have occurred:

- Maintain an airway (intubate if necessary);
- Provide oxygen;
- Administer activated charcoal;
- Give IV diazepam 0.1 to 0.3 mg/kg up to 10 mg; and
- Carefully monitor vital signs.

FACTORS AFFECTING THEOPHYLLINE EFFECTS AND CLEARANCE RATE:

Agents that increase theophylline effects:

Erythromycin, influenza vaccine, oral contraceptives, cimetidine, furosemide, verapamil.

Agents that decrease theophylline effects:

Cigarette and marijuana smoking, phenobarbital, β-adrenergic blocking agents.

Agents that increase theophylline clearance:

Cigarette and marijuana smoking, phenobarbital, high-protein diet, low-carbohydrate diet, charcoal-broiled diet, rifampin, phenytoin.

Agents that decrease theophylline clearance:

Hepatic cirrhosis, CHF, β-adrenergic blocking agents, erythromycin, cor pulmonale, oral contraceptives, cimetidine.

THEOPHYLLINE SERUM LEVELS

Target range: 8 to 20 μg/ml (recommended by the American Thoracic Society).

Desired clinical effect: maximal bronchodilation, maximal therapeutic effects.

<5 μg/ml: no effect.

5 to 10 μg/ml: mild bronchodilation, suboptimal therapeutic effects.

20 to 30 μg/ml: mild to moderate toxicity (refer to Adverse Reactions for unwanted effects).

>40 μg/ml: severe toxicity (refer to Overdosage for unwanted effects).

Specific therapeutic levels and toxic levels are highly variable between patients. An increase in the dose of theophylline may be contraindicated when a patient elicits unwanted side effects, even though a serum theophylline level is less than 8 μg/ml. In this case, a β-adrenergic agonist may be given with low-dose theophylline to produce a synergistic effect of the two drugs. On the other hand, a patient may tolerate and need a higher serum theophylline level for clinical improvement. However, a serum theophylline level greater than 30 μg/ml constitutes a medical emergency in which theophylline administration is withheld and the patient is monitored for signs of toxicity.

The loading doses of the following drugs are based on the assumption that for each 0.5 mg/kg of theophylline administered, a 1.0 μg/ml increase in serum theophylline will result. Serum theophylline levels should be monitored before and after drug administration. Any dose that is not tolerated is contraindicated.

THEOPHYLLINE

Immediate-release capsules and tablets: *Varies from 100 to 300 mg:* Bronkodyl, Elixophyllin, Somephyllin-T, generic theophylline, Slo-Phyllin, Theolair, Theophyl-225, Quibron-T-Dividose.

Liquids: *Varies from 80 mg/15 ml to 150 mg/15 ml:* generic theophylline, Asmalix, Elixomin, Elixophyllin, Lanophyllin, Lixolin, Theolair, Aquaphyllin, Slo-Phyllin, Theoclear-80, Theostat-80, Accurbron, Theon, Aerolate.

Timed-release capsules: *Varies from 50 mg to 300 mg; 12-hour timed release unless otherwise stated:* Aerolate, Bronkodyl S-R, Theophylline S.R., Elixophyllin SR, Lodrane, Slo-bid Gyrocaps, Slo-Phyllin Gyrocaps, Somophyllin-CRT, Theo-24 (24 hours), Theobid Duracaps, Theoclear L.A., Theo-Dur Sprinkle, Theophyl-SR (8 hours), Theospan-SR, Theovent Long-Acting.

Timed-release tablets: *Varies from 100 mg to 500 mg; 12-hour timed release unless otherwise stated:* Theophylline SR, Constant-T, Duraphyl, LaBid,

Quibron-T/SR, Respbid, Sustaire, Theochron, Theo-Dur (12 to 24 hours), Theolair-SR, Theo-Time, Uniphyl (12 to 24 hours).

Onset of action:	Varies; uncoated tablets 15 to 30 minutes.
Duration:	Varies, depending on route and dosage form. However, theophylline is usually given every 6 hours, unless it is administered in a timed-release capsule or tablet.
Dosage form:	As listed above.
Dosage:	
Immediate-release oral form:	*Adults:* ***PO:*** 200 to 250 mg q 6 hr. *Children:* ***PO:*** 100 mg q 6 hr.
For an acute attack:	*Adults:* 5 mg/kg initially, followed by maintenance does of 3 to 4 mg/kg q 6 hr. (May increase gradually to 6 mg/kg q 6 hr to control symptoms. *Children:* 6 mg/kg initially, followed by maintenance dose of 4 to 5 mg/kg q 6 hr.
Maintenance dosage adjustments:	*For adult nonsmokers and older adults* (>50 years): 2 to 3 mg/kg q 8 hr. *For patients with cardiac or liver disease:* 1 to 2 mg/kg q 12 hr.
Timed-release oral form:	*Adults and children:* Initial dose of 4 mg/kg q 8 to 12 hr.

Maximum daily (24 hr) oral dose:

Children <9 years:	24 mg/kg/day
Children 9 to 12 years:	20 mg/kg/day
12 to 16 years:	18 mg/kg/day
>16 years:	13 mg/kg/day or 900 mg (whichever is less)

AMINOPHYLLINE (THEOPHYLLINE ETHYLENEDIAMINE)

Immediate-release tablets: *100-mg tablets (equivalent to 79 mg theophylline), 200-mg tablets (equivalent to 158 mg theophylline):* Aminophylline (100, 200 mg), Amoline (100, 200 mg).

Oral liquid: *105 mg/5 ml (equivalent to 90 mg theophylline):* Aminophylline, Somophyllin.

Timed-release tablets: *225 mg (equivalent to 178 mg theophylline):* Phyllocontin (12 hours timed release).

Suppositories: *250 mg (equivalent to 198 mg theophylline), 500 mg (equivalent to 395 mg theophylline):* Aminophylline (250 mg, 500 mg), Truphylline (250 mg, 500 mg).

Rectal solution: *300 mg/5 ml (equivalent to 255 mg theophylline):* Somophyllin.

For IV use:

Injection: *250 mg/10 ml (equivalent to 197 mg theophylline), 500 mg/20 ml (equivalent to 394 mg theophylline), 500 mg/2 ml (equivalent to 395 mg theophylline):* Aminophylline (various).

Injection: *100 mg/100 ml plus 450 mg sodium chloride (equivalent to 78.8 mg theophylline):* Aminophylline in 0.45% sodium chloride.

Injection: *200 mg/100 ml plus 450 mg sodium chloride (equivalent to 157.6 mg theophylline):* Aminophylline in 0.45% sodium chloride.

Mode of action: Aminophylline is a composite of theophylline (79%) with ethylenediamine. Ethylenediamine enhances the solubility of the theophylline molecule. Ethylenediamine also adds to the efficacy and toxicity of theophylline. Dosages are greatly individualized and are usually based on theophylline equivalents (e.g., 100 mg of aminophylline is equal to 79 mg theophylline). Aminophylline is primarily indicated for reversal of bronchoconstriction; however, aminophylline is also indicated for use in patients who exhibit Cheyne-Stokes respirations.

Onset of action: Within 15 minutes (IV loading dose).

Duration: Varies with route and formulation.

Dosage form: As listed above.

Dosage:

Adults:

PO: For acute attack, 500 mg. Maintenance, 200 to 315 mg q 6 to 8 hr.

Rectal solution: 5 ml (255 mg theophylline) 1 to 3 times daily.

IM: 500 mg (very painful).

Children:

PO: For acute attack, 7.5 mg/kg. Maintenance, 3 to 6 mg/kg q 6 to 8 hr.

Rectal solution: 5 mg/kg q 6 hr.
Adults and children:
IV injection: For an acute attack administer a loading dose of 6 mg/kg given slowly (10 to 20 minutes), infused at a rate of no more than 25 mg/min. Reduce loading dose by 50% if patient has received theophylline within the last 24 hours. Maintenance dose: up to 0.9 mg/kg/hr by infusion. Reduce maintenance dose for patients with CHF, liver disease (0.1 to 0.2 mg/kg/hr), older patients and patients with cor pulmonale (0.3 mg/kg/hr), and otherwise healthy nonsmokers (0.5 mg/kg/hr).

DYPHYLLINE (DIHYDROXYPROPYL THEOPHYLLINE)

Immediate-release tablets: *200 mg, 400 mg:* Dyphylline (various), Dilor, Dyflex, Lufyllin, Neothylline.
Elixir: *100 mg/15 ml:* Lufyllin.
Elixir: *160 mg/15 ml:* Dilor.
Injection (IM only): *250 mg/ml:* Dyphylline (various), Dilor, Dy-Phyl-Lin, Lufyllin, Oxystat.

Mode of action: This derivative of theophylline is slightly less potent than theophylline; however, adverse reactions are less prominent. Dyphylline is an alternative drug for patients sensitive to ethylenediamine. Measurements of serum theophylline levels will not measure dyphylline levels; specific serum dyphylline levels must be used to monitor therapy.

Onset of action: Dose related, usually within 45 minutes.

Duration: Dose related, approximately 4 to 6 hours.

Dosage form: As listed above.

Dosage:
Adults:
PO: Up to 15 mg/kg qid.
IM: 250 to 500 mg; not to exceed 15 mg/kg q 6 hr. Solution must be injected slowly.
Children:
PO: 4.5 to 5.8 mg/kg bid or tid.
IM: 4.4 to 6.6 mg/kg/day in divided doses.

PROPHYLACTIC ANTIASTHMATIC AGENTS 13

PATHOPHYSIOLOGY OF BRONCHIAL ASTHMA

Bronchial asthma is a condition characterized by increased irritability of the airways by various stimuli. As one of the most common pulmonary disorders, asthma is estimated to exist in 10% of all people. No one age group, population, or sex is exempt.

An acute asthma attack (regardless of cause) is characterized by bronchospasm, mucosal edema, and excessive mucus secretion. In combination, these factors cause airway obstruction, hypoxemia, and hyperinflation. During an acute attack, respiratory distress is obvious. Dyspnea, cough with tenacious sputum production, and wheezing are present. Status asthmaticus is a life-threatening asthma attack that is refractory to conventional therapy (β_2-adrenergic drugs, theophylline). At this point, intravenous corticosteroids are required (see Chapter 14).

Also known as "reactive airway disease," bronchial asthma has two primary forms:

Atopic or extrinsic asthma: Allergic (immunologic) asthma. Approximately 50% of all asthmatics have this form of the disease. The causative agent precipitating an asthma attack is some external antigenic material. Common antigens (or allergens) include pollens, dust, smoke, perfumes, pets, or ragweed. Occasionally foods (milk, eggs, chocolate) or drugs (aspirin) may precipitate an attack.

This form of asthma involves the immune system in antigen-antibody formation. An allergic individual exposed to an antigen or allergen induces antibody formation specific to the antigen. The antibody is then *sensitized* to that particular antigen. The antibody of interest in allergic asthma is IgE (a circulating immunoglobulin). Once IgE becomes *sensitized* to a specific antigen, it attaches to the surface of the mast cell. By this action, the mast cell becomes receptive (see also Mediators Influencing Bronchomotor Tone in Chapter 2).

Re-exposure to the antigen causes a "bridging" with the antigen-specific IgE complex bound to the receptive mast cell. During this antigen-antibody reaction, an influx of calcium ions into the mast cell occurs and degranulation of the cell is provoked, thereby releasing the inflammatory mediators. In allergic individuals, release of mediators from the mast cells located in the respiratory tract mucosa produces bronchospasm, swelling of the bronchioles, and mucosal edema (i.e., an acute asthma attack).

Nonatopic or intrinsic asthma: Nonallergic (nonimmunologic) asthma. The asthma attack is precipitated either by some endogenous cause (nonallergic stimuli of unknown etiology) or in response to nonimmunologic stimuli such as infection, cold air, exercise, emotional upset, or stress.

This form of asthma does not involve the immune response; however, nonimmunologic, nonallergic stimuli still evoke mast cell degranulation, which then causes an acute asthma attack.

CROMOLYN SODIUM
INTAL, AARANE
NASALCROM (nasal solution)

MECHANISM OF ACTION AND INDICATIONS FOR USE:

Cromolyn sodium (disodium cromoglycate) inhibits the degranulation of mast cells by directly blocking the influx of calcium ions entering the mast cell; mediator release is then prevented (Fig. 13.1). For this reason, cromolyn is known as a "mast cell stabilizer."

Cromolyn does not appear to influence the antigen-antibody complex, nor does it exhibit antihistaminic, anti-inflammatory, or bronchodilator activity. The antiallergic activity of cromolyn is mainly prophylactic.

Cromolyn sodium is indicated for use to decrease the frequency and intensity of asthma attacks in both allergic and nonallergic asthma. Cromolyn sodium is also used in the treatment and prevention of allergic rhinitis and in the prevention of exercise-induced bronchospasm.

CONTRAINDICATIONS:

Hypersensitivity to cromolyn, acute asthmatic attacks, status asthmaticus.

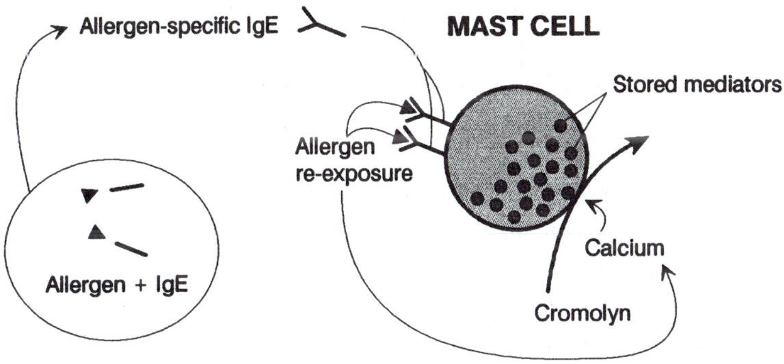

Figure 13.1. The inhibition of mast cell degranulation by cromolyn sodium.

PRECAUTIONS:

1. Cromolyn is not indicated in the treatment of an acute asthmatic attack or status asthmaticus. Cromolyn is indicated only as a prophylactic agent.
2. Cromolyn is excreted in urine and bile (feces); therefore, use with caution in patients with impaired renal or hepatic function.
3. Safety and efficacy for use in children under 5 years old and in pregnancy have not been established.
4. If cough or bronchospasm occurs, patient may not be able to continue treatment. Monitor patient for symptoms and notify physician if coughing or wheezing occurs. Prior use of a β_2-adrenergic agonist should be used if a patient develops bronchospasm and wheezing with the administration of cromolyn.

ADVERSE REACTIONS:

CNS: Dizziness, headache.

Pulmonary: Bronchospasm, wheezing, cough, laryngeal edema (rare).

GI: Nausea.

Miscellaneous: Joint swelling, abdominal pain, sneezing, nasal congestion, epistaxis, urinary frequency, throat irritation or dryness.

Allergic: Urticaria, rash, angioedema, anaphylaxis.

OVERDOSAGE:

No intervention other than medical supervision should be necessary.

Onset of action: Approximately 15 minutes.

Duration: 4 to 6 hours. Carryover effects may be as long as 2 to 3 weeks, and complete prophylactic activity may require 4 to 6 weeks.

Dosage form: ***Inhal solution:*** 20 mg/2 ml liquid ampule.
Inhal capsules: 20 mg/dry powdered capsule (to be used with Spinhaler).
MDI: 800 µg/inhalation.
Nasal solution: 40 mg/ml (4%)

Dosage: *Adults:*
Ampule for nebulization or dry powdered capsules:
1 ampule via SVN or 1 capsule via Spinhaler inhaled 4 times daily given at regular intervals.
Children:
Ampule for nebulization:
for children ≥ 2 years old; same dose as for adult.
Dry powdered capsules:
for children > 5 years old; same dose as for adult.
For prevention of exercise-induced bronchospasm: Inhale one capsule via Spinhaler or 1 ampule via SVN no more than 60 minutes prior to exercise.
Adults:
MDI: 2 metered sprays inhaled 4 times daily, given at regular intervals. Not to exceed this dose.
Children:
MDI: for children ≥ 5 years old; same dose as for adult.
For prevention of exercise-induced bronchospasm or for exposure to cold air or environmental agents: 2 metered dose sprays 10 to 15 minutes, but not more than 60 minutes, prior to exercise or external stimulus.
Nasal Spray: *Adults and children 6 years and older:* 1 spray in each nostril 3 to 6 times per day, given at regular intervals.

KETOTIFEN
ZADITEN

Ketotifen is a drug currently under investigation as an antiasthmatic agent. Ketotifen exhibits the same pharmacologic activities as cromolyn: antihistaminic and antianaphylactic activity. However, ketotifen has the added advantage of oral administration.

Clinical studies have shown that 1 mg of ketotifen given orally twice daily has the same effect as 20 mg of cromolyn given four times daily. As with cromolyn, the complete prophylactic activity of ketotifen requires approximately 4 to 6 weeks. However, there are a few documented case studies in which ketotifen failed to provide prophylaxis in adults with intrinsic (nonallergic) asthma and in exercise-induced bronchospasm in children with asthma.

The side effects of ketotifen include sedation, drowsiness, headache, weight gain, dry mouth, and dizziness. Overdosage symptoms include mild abdominal pain, confusion, bradycardia, hyperexcitability, tachycardia, dyspnea, tachypnea, cyanosis, convulsions, and unconsciousness.

While ketotifen may not replace established antiasthmatic drugs, it is a potential alternative in the prophylaxis of asthma. Ketotifen is already available in Britain and Europe. Pending further approval in the United States, Sandoz plans to market the drug under the name of Zaditen.

NEDOCROMIL SODIUM
TILADE

Nedocromil sodium is another antiasthmatic drug currently undergoing investigation. As with cromolyn, nedocromil has the ability to inhibit mediator release from mast cells.

Approximate dosage is 4 mg in MDI form administered two to four times daily. Adverse effects include headache, dizziness, unpleasant taste, nausea, and vomiting.

Various clinical studies have shown that with the use of nedocromil, patients are effectively able to decrease the need for (but not totally eliminate) bronchodilators and inhaled corticosteroids.

Anti-Inflammatory Glucocorticosteroids 14

Adrenocorticosteroids are naturally occurring hormones secreted by the adrenal cortex. These corticosteroids are classified into three groups according to their chemical structure and major physiological effects: *(a)* glucocorticosteroids (anti-inflammatory and immunosuppressant actions), *(b)* mineralocorticosteroids (maintain water and electrolyte balance), and *(c)* sex hormones. Of main concern to the practitioner are the glucocorticosteroids used in respiratory care, of which the synthetic derivative of hydrocortisone is the prototype, owing to its powerful efficacy as an anti-inflammatory agent.

Review of Glucocorticosteroids

The hypothalamus contains corticotropin-releasing hormone (CRH) which, when released, travels through a portal system of blood vessels to the pituitary gland. Once at the pituitary gland, CRH stimulates the pituitary corticotrophs to secrete adrenocorticotrophic hormone (ACTH). ACTH then mediates the synthesis and release of glucocorticoids (primarily hydrocortisone [cortisol] at the adrenal cortex). The degree of ACTH stimulation at the adrenal cortex is a direct factor of plasma cortisol levels. Elevated plasma levels of cortisol decrease ACTH secretion, and, likewise, reduced plasma levels of cortisol increase the secretion of ACTH. Externally administered corticosteroids suppress the normal mechanism of the hypothalamus-pituitary-adrenal (HPA) transport system. This is why the dosage of corticosteroids, when administered for more than two weeks, need to be gradually tapered, allowing the HPA transport mechanism to return to its normal functioning level, otherwise an adrenal crisis may occur and may potentiate the disease state.

MECHANISM OF ACTION AND INDICATIONS FOR USE:

The pharmacologic actions of glucocorticosteroids are varied; the major actions pertaining to respiratory care are summarized below:

1. *Anti-inflammatory action*—Inhibits the formation and release of inflammatory mediators by interfering with the degranulation of the mast cell.
2. *Increased sympathomimetic effects*—Inhibits COMT from metabolizing catecholamines.
3. *Enhanced ciliary transport*—Decreases mucus secretion by altering mucus composition.
4. *Enhanced sympathomimetic responsiveness*—Indirectly stimulates cAMP production by restoring responsiveness to β-adrenergic stimulation.
5. *Improved general sense of well-being.*

For treatment in chest diseases, glucocorticosteroids are indicated for use in acute and chronic asthmatic attacks (only if conventional therapy has failed: β-adrenergic agents, theophylline, avoidance of provoking stimuli), status asthmaticus, severe COPD, hypersensitivity pneumonitis, active interstitial lung disease, neonatal respiratory distress syndrome, adult respiratory distress syndrome (controversial), aspiration pneumonitis, and allergic rhinitis. Systemic administration of steroids is indicated for an acute asthma attack and status asthmaticus, while aerosolized steroids are primarily used for control of severe asthma and in patients with chronic asthma. Table 14.1 lists the advantages and disadvantages of systemic and aerosol administration of steroids.

CONTRAINDICATIONS:

Hypersensitivity to any of the drug's ingredients, systemic fungal infections (due to their immunosuppressant actions corticosteroids mask the symptoms of infection), patients with psychoses, peptic ulcer, acute glomerulonephritis, herpes simplex of the eye, severe diabetes mellitus.

PRECAUTIONS:

1. These agents are not direct bronchodilators; therefore, they are not indicated for the rapid relief of bronchospasm.
2. Aerosol corticosteroids have less HPA suppression effects than systemic corticosteroids; however, if recommended dosages are exceeded (>1000 μg/day), the HPA transport mechanism may be influenced.
3. Use with caution in pregnancy. Use only if the benefits outweigh the potential risk to the fetus.

Table 14.1.
Comparison of Oral and Aerosol Steroids for Asthma[a]

	Oral	Aerosol
ADVANTAGES OF AEROSOL FORMULATIONS		
Development of Cushing's syndrome with optimal dose	Yes	No
Suppression of HPA mechanism	Yes	No (doses of <1000 μg/day).
Development of a steroid-dependent state	High risk	Low risk
Local therapeutic effects	No	Yes
ADVANTAGES OF ORAL FORMULATIONS		
Ease of administration	Simple	Complex
Dosage schedules	Well dictated	Not well established
Cost	Inexpensive	Expensive
Hazards of therapy	Well documented	All hazards not fully known
Potential improper use (e.g., as a "bronchodilator")	Medium risk	High risk
Used for status asthmaticus	Yes	No
Risk of superinfection	Moderate	Greater risk
Local airway reaction	No	Hoarseness Coughing Throat irritation

[a]Adapted from Ziment I. Respiratory pharmacology and therapeutics. Philadelphia: WB Saunders, 1978.

4. Prolonged therapy may cause a Cushing-like syndrome (moon face, edema, "hump" back) with subsequent adrenal insufficiency.
5. When tapering dosages, monitor patient for steroid withdrawal syndrome: anorexia, nausea, vomiting, lethargy, headache, hypotension.
6. Administer PO forms with food to minimize ulcer activity.
7. To minimize side effects, local administration is preferred over systemic therapy when indicated.
8. Long-term steroid therapy requires the smallest dose that will produce the desired effects.
9. Corticosteroids are indicated only when the patient has failed to respond

to conventional therapy (e.g., sympathomimetic bronchodilators, theophylline, and other nonsteroid medications).

10. Use with caution in patients with renal disease or impairment; edema may occur.

ADVERSE REACTIONS: SYSTEMIC CORTICOSTEROIDS

Suppression of the HPA system and the adrenal cortex.

Fluid and Electrolyte Imbalance: Sodium and fluid retention, edema, hypokalemia, metabolic alkalosis.

Cardiovascular: Fat embolism, thromboembolism, cardiac arrhythmias, syncope, hypertension.

GI: Pancreatitis, abdominal distention, nausea, vomiting, increased appetite, weight gain, peptic ulcer, perforation of the small and large bowel.

CNS: Headache, vertigo, insomnia, restlessness, seizures, mood swings, depression, euphoria.

Musculoskeletal: Muscle wasting, muscle pain, osteoporosis, delayed wound healing.

Miscellaneous: Growth suppression, obesity, Cushingoid appearance, hyperglycemia, diabetes, and immunosuppression.

ADVERSE REACTIONS: AEROSOL CORTICOSTEROIDS

Local: Throat irritation, hoarseness, dry mouth, coughing, oropharyngeal fungal infection (*Candida albicans* or *Aspergillus niger*) (rinsing and gargling after MDI administration may reduce the incidence of this infection.)

Systemic: Suppression of the HPA mechanism (with excessive doses, >1000 μg/day).

Other: Bronchospasm (rare), rash (rare).

AEROSOL CORTICOSTEROIDS

BECLOMETHASONE DIPROPIONATE
BECLOVENT, VANCERIL

Mode of action: Rapidly absorbed long-acting anti-inflammatory agent. Usage may permit a gradual decrease in the dosage of the systemic corticosteroid. Sometimes used as an alternative to cromolyn sodium.

Plasma half-life: 15 hours.

Dosage form: *MDI:* 42 μg/inhalation.

Dosage: *Adults:*
2 inhalations 3 to 4 times daily. Not to exceed 20 inhalations daily.
Children:
6 to 12 years old:
1 to 2 inhalations tid or qid. Not to exceed 10 inhalations daily.

DEXAMETHASONE SODIUM PHOSPHATE
DECRADRON PHOSPHATE RESPIHALER

Mode of action: Rapidly absorbed anti-inflammatory agent.
Plasma half-life: 5 hours.
Dosage form: *MDI:* 84 μg/inhalation.
Dosage: *Adults:*
3 inhalations tid or qid. Maximum dosage: 3 inhalations per dose, 12 inhalations per day.
Children:
2 inhalations tid or qid. Maximum dosage: 2 inhalations per dose, 8 inhalations per day.

FLUNISOLIDE
AEROBID

Mode of action: Rapidly absorbed anti-inflammatory agent. Several days may be required for the full therapeutic effects to occur.
Plasma half-life: 1.6 hours.
Dosage form: *MDI:* 250 μg/inhalation.
Dosage: *Adults:*
2 inhalations bid (morning and evening). Total daily dose, 1 mg. Not to exceed 4 inhalations twice daily.
Children:
6 to 15 years old: 2 inhalations bid.

TRIAMCINOLONE ACETONIDE
AZMACORT

Mode of action: Intermediate-acting anti-inflammatory agent. Full therapeutic effects may be noted in 5 to 10 days, with onset of therapeutic activity noted in 1 to 3 days.

Plasma half-life: ½ to 1 hour.
Dosage form: ***MDI:*** 100 μg/inhalation.
Dosage: *Adults:*
2 inhalations tid or qid. Not to exceed 16 inhalations per day.
Children:
6 to 12 years old:
1 to 2 inhalations tid or qid. Not to exceed 12 inhalations per day.

BUDESONIDE (INVESTIGATIONAL)

Mode of action: Rapidly absorbed anti-inflammatory agent.
Plasma half-life: 2 to 2.8 hours.
Dosage form: ***MDI:*** 50 μg/inhalation.
Dosage: *Adults:*
400 to 1600 μg/day in 2 to 4 doses.
Children:
200 to 400 μg/day in 2 to 4 doses.

COMMONLY USED INTRAVENOUS AND ORAL CORTICOSTEROIDS

DEXAMETHASONE
DECADRON, HEXADROL

Mode of action: Potent, long-acting anti-inflammatory agent. Lacks sodium retaining activity with low to moderate doses. Dexamethasone is rapidly absorbed after oral administration.
Plasma half-life: Males, 3.4 hours; Females, 2.4 hours.
Dosage form: ***PO:*** 0.25-, 0.5-, 0.75-, 1-, 1.5-, 2-, 4-, 6-mg tablets.
0.5 mg/5 ml elixir.
0.5 mg/5 ml oral solution.
IV: 4, 10, 20, 24 mg/ml.
Dosage: ***PO, IV:*** Initially 0.75 to 9 mg/day given bid or qid.
For cerebral edema: Initially 10 mg IV, then 4 mg IM q 6 hr.

HYDROCORTISONE SODIUM SUCCINATE
SOLU-CORTEF

Mode of action: Relatively short-acting anti-inflammatory agent. Normal daily secretion of hydrocortisone in humans is 10 to 25 mg. Normal plasma level is 5 to 30 μg/100 ml. Used in the treatment of status asthmaticus and other acute chest diseases.

Plasma half-life: 80 to 118 minutes.

Onset of action: <60 minutes. Peak action occurs in approximately 5 hours. Excreted within 12 hours.

Dosage form: ***IV, IM solution:*** 100 mg, 250 mg, 500 mg, 1000 mg.

Dosage: Initially, may give up to 500 mg/day.
Loading dose: Severe asthma, 4 mg/kg or 300 mg. Then 1 mg/kg q 1 hr.
Maintenance dose: 0.5 mg/kg/hr by continuous infusion or 100 to 200 mg q 3 to 6 hr.

METHYLPREDNISOLONE
SOLU-MEDROL (IV), MEDROL (ORAL)

Mode of action: Potent intermediate-acting anti-inflammatory agent. Minimal sodium retaining activity. Alternate drug to hydrocortisone for hypersensitivity reactions, status asthmaticus, aspiration pneumonitis, ARDS.

Plasma half-life: 78 to 188 minutes.

Onset of action: Slow, 12 to 24 hours.

Duration: Long, up to one week.

Dosage form: ***IV, IM solution:*** 40, 125, 500, 1000 mg per vial. 2000 mg (powder).
PO: 2-, 4-, 8-, 16-, 24-, 32-mg tablets.

Dosage: ***PO:*** Initially 4 to 48 mg/day.
IV, IM: Initially 10 to 40 mg/day.
Loading dose: Severe asthma, 0.8 mg/kg.

PREDNISONE
ORASONE, DELTASONE, METICORTEN

Mode of action: Intermediate-acting anti-inflammatory agent. Prednisone is one of the more commonly used steroids and is 3 to 5 times as potent as hydrocortisone. Moderate fluid retention activity. Prednisone is metabolized to its active form prednisolone in the liver (oral prednisolone is substituted in patients with liver disease).

Plasma half-life: Approximately 60 minutes.

Dosage form:	***PO:*** 1-, 2.5-, 5-, 10-, 20-, 25-, 50-mg tablets. 5 mg/5 ml, 5 mg/ml oral solution. 5 mg/5 ml syrup.
Dosage:	Highly individualized. Initially, 5 to 60 mg per day. *Loading dose:* Mild asthma attack, 40 to 60 mg. *Maintenance dose:* 20 mg q 4 to 6 hr. Gradually decrease dose to qd or qod.

PREDNISOLONE
DELTA-CORTEF, STERANE, HYDELTRASOL

Mode of action:	Essentially the same action as prednisone. Prednisolone is also one of the more commonly used corticosteroids for allergic and inflammatory conditions.
Plasma half-life:	115 to 212 minutes.
Dosage form:	***PO:*** 5-mg tablets. 15 mg/5 ml, 5 mg/5 ml syrup. ***IV, IM:*** 20 mg/ml.
Dosage:	Highly individualized. ***PO, IV, IM:*** Initially 4 to 60 mg/day.

Inhalational Mucolytic Agents and Surface-Active Agents 15

Methods of Mucolytics

There are several known methods of altering the biochemical nature of mucus. Each method exemplifies a specific mode of action that tends either to lessen the viscosity of mucus, to control the production of mucus, or to liquefy secretions to facilitate bronchial hygiene.

The first method presented in this chapter lowers the viscosity of mucus by replacing the disulfide bond (SS) of the mucoprotein with its own free sulfhydryl (SH) group (acetylcysteine). The second method presented enhances an increased topical pH in the lung mucosa, which weakens the saccharide side chains of the mucoprotein, thereby decreasing mucus viscosity (sodium bicarbonate). The third method humidifies and liquefies pulmonary secretions by directly adding liquid to the tracheobronchial tree (wetting agents). Finally, the fourth method presented invades and destroys the polypeptide core of the mucoprotein structure and/or DNA, thereby lessening the viscosity of mucus (proteolytic enzymes). Also included in this chapter is propylene glycol (disrupts the mucoprotein by breaking the hydrogen bonds). To date, only acetylcysteine is approved by the FDA for use as an aerosol mucolytic. The surface-active agents (alcohol and surfactant) concludes the chapter.

ACETYLCYSTEINE
MUCOMYST, MUCOSAL

MECHANISM OF ACTION AND INDICATIONS FOR USE:

Acetylcysteine, a compound $C_5H_9NO_3S$, is a derivative of the naturally occurring amino acid L-cysteine. Acetylcysteine replaces the disulfide (SS) bonds of mucoproteins with its own free sulfhydryl (SH) group, thus lowering the viscosity of mucus (Fig. 15.1). The mucolytic action of acetylcysteine significantly increases with increasing pH (7.0 to 9.0).

Acetylcysteine is indicated as adjuvant therapy for tenacious, viscid, or inspissated mucus in disease states such as chronic emphysema, acute and chronic bronchitis, tuberculosis, bronchiectasis, pneumonia, tracheobronchitis, and atelectasis due to mucus obstruction. It is also indicated for pulmonary complications of cystic fibrosis, tracheostomy care, and those associated with surgery. Acetylcysteine is also used for diagnostic bronchial studies such as bronchograms, bronchospirometry, and bronchial wedge catheterization.

In acetaminophen poisoning, acetylcysteine is indicated as an antidote to lessen hepatic injury that may occur.

CONTRAINDICATIONS:

Hypersensitivity to acetylcysteine, patients at risk of gastric hemorrhage.

PRECAUTIONS:

1. After the administration of acetylcysteine, there may be an increased volume of liquefied bronchial secretions. In patients who demonstrate a weak or ineffective cough, tracheal suctioning may be necessary.
2. If bronchospasm occurs, acetylcysteine should be discontinued or be given concurrently with a bronchodilator (preferred choice).

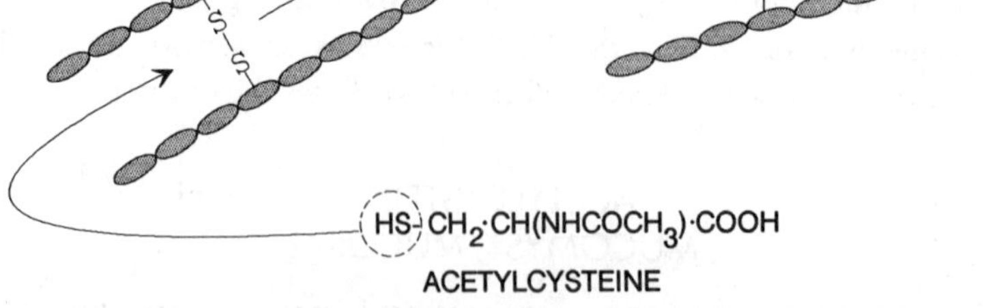

Figure 15.1. Acetylcysteine effects on the mucoprotein structure. (Adapted from Ziment I. Respiratory pharmacology and therapeutics. Philadelphia: WB Saunders, 1978.)

3. Acetylcysteine may inactivate a number of antibiotics (especially penicillin type drugs). Therefore, these drugs should not be given concomitantly.
4. Acetylcysteine produces a characteristic foul-smelling odor that is caused by the liberation of hydrogen sulfide.
5. Acetlycysteine adversely reacts with rubber, copper, and iron. Opened vials should be stored in a refrigerator and discarded in 96 hours.

ADVERSE REACTIONS:

Miscellaneous: Nausea, vomiting.

Pulmonary: Bronchospasm (especially with asthmatics), coughing, irritation of mucosa.

Persistent use: Rhinitis, laryngitis, tracheitis, severe hoarseness, hemoptysis, stomatitis, rhinorrhea.

Onset of action:	<1 minute.
Peak effects:	5 to 10 minutes.
Dosage form:	***Inhal solution:*** 10%, 20%.
Dosage:	***Recommended dosage:*** 3 to 5 ml of 20% solution equally diluted with Sterile Water for Injection, U.S.P., or with normal saline given 3 to 4 times daily via nebulization; or 6 to 10 ml of 10% solution (undiluted) 3 to 4 times daily via nebulization. *Direct installation into the lungs of an intubated patient:* 1 to 2 ml of 10% or 20% solution. *For diagnostic bronchograms:* 1 to 2 ml of 20% solution or 2 to 4 ml of 10% solution, given prior to or during the procedure. *For acetaminophen overdosage:* Loading dose, 140 mg/kg. Maintenance dose, 70 mg/kg for a total of 17 doses.

SODIUM 2-MERCAPTOETHANE SULFONATE
MISTABRON

Mistabron is a mucolytic agent with actions and effects similar to acetylcysteine. Available in a 20% solution, Mistabron is currently used only in Great Britain.

SODIUM BICARBONATE

MECHANISM OF ACTION AND INDICATIONS FOR USE:

Sodium bicarbonate ($NaHCO_3$) is a weak base (pH 7.4 to 8.5) that, when inhaled, directly increases bronchial pH. This results in weakening and thereby rupturing the saccharide side chain of the mucoprotein structure. This then produces a decrease in mucus viscosity. Sodium bicarbonate may be combined with other drugs for immediate use and may be used as a diluent for acetylcysteine to potentiate the effects of acetylcysteine, whose effects are enhanced in the alkaline environment.

CONTRAINDICATIONS:
Use with caution if delivering large amounts and higher concentrations. May cause hypernatremia or metabolic alkalosis.

ADVERSE REACTIONS:
Adverse reactions are noted only when solutions of >2% are used. May cause bronchomucosal and oropharyngeal irritation. Concurrent administration of bronchodilators may be used to prevent bronchospasm.

Dosage: Sodium bicarbonate is available for inhalation in concentrations of 1.4, 5, and 7.5%. Recommended strength for less irritating effects is equal dilution of the 5% solution, producing a 2.5% solution. For nebulization, 2 to 5 ml q 4 to 8 hours. For intratracheal installation, 5 to 10 ml as needed. Alkalosis may occur if drug is overused.

Note: When administering sodium bicarbonate concomitantly with a bronchodilator, the solution must be mixed immediately prior to administration and any remaining solution must be discarded. In an alkaline environment, such as that with sodium bicarbonate, bronchodilators are inactivated. Color changes of the drug occur owing to a breakdown of products (sputum may then have a red tinge when expectorated).

WETTING AGENTS

STERILE DISTILLED WATER: Aerosolized inhaled water is partially absorbed into the cell, owing to the cell's diffusion gradient. The remainder of solution that is not absorbed into the cell hydrates secretions, thereby liquefying secretions and promoting expectoration.

Sterile distilled water is indicated to humidify dry inspired gases, and especially to provide humidification when the upper airway is bypassed.

NORMAL SALINE: Isotonic solution (0.9% of NaCl) that denotes the same tonicity as body fluids. There is no diffusion of water into or out of the cell membrane, owing to the equal tension generated on both sides of the semipermeable cell membrane. Because there is no net flow of water across the cell membrane, the inhaled aerosol particles tend to remain stable in size throughout the tracheobronchial tree and impact in the more distal airways. Normal saline minimizes tracheobronchial irritation and is less irritating than water.

Normal saline is indicated for use as a diluent with bronchodilators and for use by itself to liquefy secretions through direct instillation of the lungs in the intubated patient.

HYPERTONIC SALINE: A solution of NaCl that is greater than 0.9%. Hypertonic saline has a greater osmotic pressure than body fluids and therefore causes diffusion of water out of the cell. This may generate cellular dehydration and overhydration of the intracellular space. Due to the influx of cellular water, the inhaled aerosol particles tend to increase in size throughout the tracheobronchial tree and impact in the upper and middle portions of the airway.

Hypertonic saline is primarily indicated to stimulate a productive cough and for sputum induction. This solution is very irritating to the airway and may cause bronchospasm.

HYPOTONIC SALINE: A solution of NaCl that is less than 0.9% (usually 0.45% of NaCl). Due to the cell's diffusion gradient, hypotonic saline solution is absorbed into and through the cellular membrane, therefore the inhaled aerosol particles become smaller throughout the tracheobronchial tree and tend to impact in the more distal airways.

Hypotonic saline solution is generally indicated when other more irritating solutions are contraindicated or for those patients on restricted sodium intake. This concentration of NaCl seems to be less irritating to the airway and least affects airway resistance.

CONTRAINDICATIONS:

Large amounts of saline and water solutions are contraindicated in patients with congestive heart failure and in neonates. Large amounts of these solutions may lead to fluid overload and peripheral edema. In patients with sodium restriction, care should be taken not to exceed the daily limitation through the administration of saline solutions. When total electrolyte administration is contraindicated, saline solutions should not be given.

ADVERSE REACTIONS:

Miscellaneous: Fluid overload, edema (primarily noted with hypertonic saline solutions and in neonates).

Pulmonary: Bronchospasm, coughing, swelling of secretions that may result in airway occlusion, atelectasis (primarily noted with hypertonic saline solutions).

Some patients may not be able to tolerate the "salty" taste of hypertonic saline solutions. Gagging, choking, nausea, or vomiting may occur.

PROTEOLYTIC ENZYMES

MECHANISM OF ACTION:
Proteolytic enzymes (such as pancreatic dornase) have been noted to decrease the viscosity of purulent and nonpurulent secretions by attacking either the polypeptide core of the mucoprotein structure or DNA (a component of purulent sputum responsible for its viscosity) or both. Because these enzymes are expensive to use, have a high toxic potential, are irritating to the respiratory tract, and may produce antibodies, they are not useful as inhalational mucolytic agents.

PROPYLENE GLYCOL

MECHANISM OF ACTION AND INDICATIONS FOR USE:
Propylene glycol is a hygroscopic agent that absorbs moisture and resists dehydration. Propylene glycol disrupts the mucoprotein structure by breaking hydrogen bonds. It also stabilizes aerosol particles by preventing evaporation, thereby improving distal deposition in the airway.

Propylene glycol (2 to 25%) may be indicated when other inhalational therapy produces less than desired effects.

CONTRAINDICATIONS:
Propylene glycol inhibits the growth of the *Mycobacterium tuberculosis* species in sputum, therefore it is contraindicated in patients suspected of this disease.

ADVERSE REACTIONS:
Excessive doses may cause coughing and irritation of the proximal airways.

Dosage: Nebulize 1 to 2 ml of 2% solution concurrently with a bronchodilator or another mucokinetic agent. For very viscous secretions: Nebulize 10 to 20% of propylene glycol solution for 20 minutes.

SURFACE-ACTIVE AGENTS

ALCOHOL
ETHANOL, ETHYL ALCOHOL

MECHANISM OF ACTION AND INDICATIONS FOR USE:
Alcohol is a surface active agent that has the ability to lower the surface tension of bubbly, frothy respiratory tract secretions. By lowering the surface tension of these secretions, a much smaller volume is noted with improvement of ventilation. Ethyl alcohol may be indicated for use in acute pulmonary edema;

however, the use is rare owing to the advent of more sophisticated drugs (cardiotonics, diuretics).

CONTRAINDICATIONS:

Patients on Antabuse therapy.

ADVERSE REACTIONS:

Pulmonary: Lung mucosa irritation, bronchospasm.
Other: Slightly intoxicated state, local dehydration.

Dosage: Ethyl alcohol: Nebulize 5 to 15 ml of 30% to 50% solution (short treatments are recommended).

Note: Do not use isopropyl or denatured alcohol. Tyloxapol (Alevaire) and sodium ethasulfate (Tergemist) are no longer recommended for use in the control of pulmonary secretions due to the lack of proof of efficacy as stated by the FDA.

EXOGENOUS SURFACTANTS

The synthesis of surfactant normally occurs within the lung by alveolar type II cells. Liberated surfactant reduces the surface tension of the alveoli (keeps alveoli open and stable), thereby enhancing alveolar elasticity and gas exchange.

70% of deaths among preterm newborns are due to the immature lungs failing to produce sufficient quantities of surfactant. Synonymous names associated with this condition include surfactant deficiency disease (SDD), respiratory distress syndrome (RDS), and hyaline membrane disease (HMD).

Surfactant replacement therapy is a relatively new area of study, however; early results indicate that a single dose of exogenous surfactant dramatically improves lung function in the preterm newborn.

The most promising, beneficial results have been noted with biologically derived extracts (see Appendix C). Effective dosage range: 60 to 120 mg given as a bolus (3 to 5 ml) through the ET tube.

16 Respiratory Depressants

Respiratory depressants, as the name implies, depress respirations and suppress ventilatory drive. The degree of depression of these drugs is directly dose related. Therefore, the dose given should be the minimum that is consistent with therapeutic efficacy. The major categories of respiratory depressants that may profoundly affect respiration are of two types: the sedative-hypnotic agents and the narcotic analgesics. A brief summary of miscellaneous respiratory depressants concludes the chapter.

To fully understand the pharmacologic actions of these agents and of respiratory stimulants (Chapter 17), a brief review of the central nervous system (CNS) is presented.

Review of the Central Nervous System

The CNS is composed of two subsystems: the brain and the spinal cord. The spinal cord is composed of nerve fibers that serve to relay information from all body areas to the brain and then conduct the messages from the brain to all body areas.

The brain consists of three primary divisions: the forebrain, the midbrain, and the hindbrain (Fig. 16.1). The forebrain is composed of two major subdivisions: the cerebrum and the diencephalon. An external layer of gray matter, the cerebral cortex, covers the cerebrum. The cerebral cortex consists of 10 to 14 billion neurons and is responsible for regulating bodily functions and activities such as skeletal muscle movement, hearing, speech, vision, memory, learning, and discrimination of pain, temperature, and touch. The functions and activities listed above may be profoundly affected by drugs that exert their influence on cortical activity.

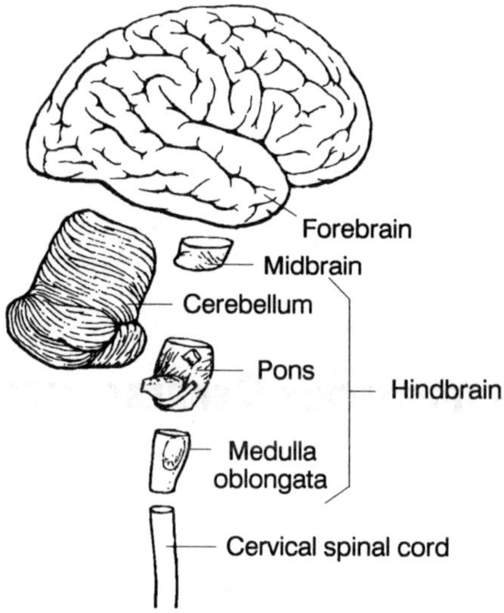

Figure 16.1. The primary divisions of the brain. Various parts of the brain have been separated to show detail.

The diencephalon of the forebrain contains the thalamus and the hypothalamus. The hypothalamus regulates visceral activities innervated by both the sympathetic and parasympathetic divisions of the autonomic nervous system. The hypothalamus is also the primary regulating center for endocrine gland secretion, body temperature, the sleeping-waking mechanisms, behavior and emotional responses, and arterial blood pressure. It contains an extensive network of neurons that connect not only with the autonomic centers but also with the thalamus and the cerebral cortex.

The thalamus, which composes the bulk of the diencephalon, is an important relay center for impulse conduction from all body parts to the cerebral cortex. It functions to sort incoming sensory messages from the periphery and then relay these messages to the cerebral cortex. The activities of the thalamus are in part controlled by the state of consciousness and crude awareness. Drugs that stimulate or depress the activities of the thalamus alter the relay of impulse transmission to the cerebral cortex.

The midbrain serves as a conduction pathway to higher brain centers and also as a reflex center for visual, auditory, and postural reflexes.

The hindbrain consists of the cerebellum, the pons, and the medulla oblongata. The pons is located between the midbrain and the medulla and, like the midbrain, the pons serves as a conduction pathway to the higher brain centers. The lower portion of the pons contains neurons that assist in the regulation of respiration and is known as the secondary respiratory coordinating center, with the medulla being the primary respiratory coordinating center.

The medulla oblongata, in addition to being a conduction pathway, also contains the body's vital centers such as the cardiac center (regulates the rate of the heart beat), the vasomotor center (constricts or dilates blood vessels), and the respiratory center (regulates rate and depth of breathing). Drugs that affect the medulla may profoundly alter any one or more of these vital centers.

The cerebellum is attached to the brain stem (midbrain, pons, medulla oblongata) and the spinal cord by three paired bundles of nerve fibers, the cerebellar peduncles. The cerebellum serves primarily to coordinate involuntary muscular activity and muscle tone.

Located throughout the brain stem, extending from the medulla to the lower portion of the thalamus, are nuclei that run in various directions. These nuclei compose the reticular formation (Fig. 16.2). Stimulation of this system results in the activation of the cerebral cortex, producing a state of alertness and attention. The upper portion of the formation plus its pathway to the thalamus and the cerebral cortex is denoted as the reticular activating system (RAS). Drugs that depress (sedate) or those that stimulate (enhance consciousness, alertness) act in part on the RAS.

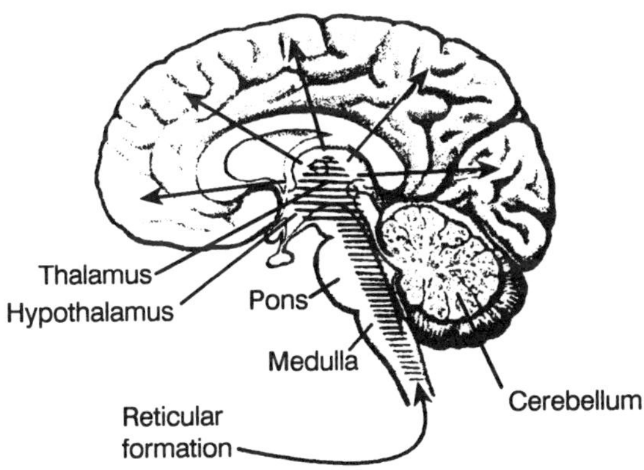

Figure 16.2. Diagram of the reticular formation, radiating from the brain stem to the cortical regions.

SEDATIVE-HYPNOTIC AGENTS

BARBITURATES

MECHANISM OF ACTION AND INDICATIONS FOR USE:
Barbiturates interfere with the relay of sensory impulses to the cerebral cortex by inhibiting the ascending impulse conduction in the reticular formation. Barbiturates induce all levels of CNS divergence from mild sedation to deep coma. All barbiturates also depress the medullary respiratory center, which results in a diminished respiratory drive. The degree of respiratory depression and CNS depression is primarily dose related.

Barbiturates are classified as long-acting, intermediate-acting, short-acting, or ultrashort-acting according to their onset of action and duration of effect.

Barbiturates are indicated for use as treatment in insomnia, as preoperative agents to reduce anxiety or fear, as aids to facilitate anesthesia, and as anticonvulsant agents.

CONTRAINDICATIONS:
Barbiturate sensitivity, liver disease, impaired renal function, patients with severe respiratory distress, respiratory disease in which dyspnea, obstruction, or cor pulmonale is present, acute or chronic pain.

PRECAUTIONS:
1. Barbiturates are habit forming. With continued use, tolerance and psychological and physical dependence may occur.
2. Use with caution in patients who have suicidal or drug histories or who are mentally depressed.
3. Use with caution in elderly patients, debilitated patients, and children (increased adverse reactions may occur).
4. Rapid IV administration may cause respiratory depression, apnea, laryngospasm, and severe hypotension.

ADVERSE REACTIONS:
CNS: Somnolence, agitation, confusion, ataxia, vertigo, CNS depression, lethargy, nervousness, anxiety, delirium.

Pulmonary: Hypoventilation, respiratory depression, apnea, laryngospasm, bronchospasm.

Cardiovascular: Bradycardia, hypotension, syncope.

GI: Nausea, vomiting, constipation, diarrhea, epigastric pain.

Other: Injection into or near peripheral nerves may produce permanent neurological deficit.

Hypersensitivity: Skin rash, angioneurotic edema, serum sickness.
Acute intoxification: Unsteady walk, slurred speech, confusion, irritability, insomnia.

OVERDOSAGE:

1 g oral dose produces serious poisoning.
2 to 10 g may cause death.

CNS and respiratory depression may progress to Cheyne-Stokes respirations along with tachycardia, hypotension, decreased body temperature, and coma. Shock syndrome may occur, which is manifested by apnea, circulatory collapse, respiratory arrest, and possible death. With extreme overdosage, a "flat" EEG may result, which is reversible if hypoxic damage has not occurred.

Pneumonia, pulmonary edema, cardiac arrhythmias, CHF, and renal failure are possible complications to barbiturate overdose.

Treatment consists of providing supportive care, maintaining an airway, intubating with assisted ventilation if necessary, and monitoring of vital signs and fluid balance. Emesis may be induced if patient has not lost consciousness, with care taken to prevent aspiration. If renal function is normal, forced diuresis may be induced. In severe barbiturate overdose, hemodialysis may be necessary. Table 16.1 lists the barbiturates.

BENZODIAZEPINES

MECHANISM OF ACTION AND INDICATIONS FOR USE:

Benzodiazepines are more commonly the drugs of choice used for sedative or hypnotic effects due to their efficacy and safety as demonstrated by considerable clinical documentation and experience. Benzodiazepines exert their effect on subcortical levels of the CNS—primarily on the limbic system (emotional and behavioral responses) and on the reticular formation. However, benzodiazepines do not relatively affect the cerebral cortex as do the barbiturates. Benzodiazepines also directly facilitate the actions of γ-aminobutyric acid (GABA). GABA is a major inhibitory neurotransmitter located at presynaptic and/or postsynaptic neurons at various levels in the brain. The results produced include antianxiety effects, muscle relaxation, sedative or hypnotic effects, and anticonvulsant effects. The benzodiazepines exert minimal effects on the medullary respiratory center, which makes them safer to use than the barbiturates.

Benzodiazepines are indicated for use for the management of anxiety disorders, as hypnotics, as anticonvulsants, as muscle relaxants, for the

Table 16.1.
The Barbiturates

Barbiturate	Oral Dose[a] Sedative	Hypnotic	Onset	Duration
	mg	*mg*	*min*	*hr*
Long-acting			60	10–12
Phenobarbital	30–120	100–320		
Mephobarbital	90–400	—		
Intermediate-acting			45–60	6–8
Amobarbital	30–480	65–200		
Aprobarbital	120	40–160		
Butabarbital	45–120	50–100		
Talbutal	60–180	120		
Short-acting			10–15	3–4
Secobarbital	—	100		
Pentobarbital	40–120	100		
	Injection range			
Ultrashort-acting			<1	½
Thiopental sodium	2–3 ml of 2.5% solution			
Thiamylal sodium	3–4 ml of 2.5% solution			
Methohexital sodium	5–12 ml of 1% solution			

[a]Total daily dose, given in 2 to 4 divided doses.

management of acute alcohol withdrawal, and as sedation for ventilator patients.

CONTRAINDICATIONS:

Hypersensitivity to benzodiazepines, psychoses, acute alcoholic intoxication, patients in shock or coma with depression of vital signs.

PRECAUTIONS:

1. Use with caution in patients with liver and/or renal disease (dosage may need to be reduced).
2. Continued use may lead to dependence.
3. Owing to the potentiation of adverse reactions use with caution in the elderly, patients with limited pulmonary reserve, the very ill, and children.
4. Avoid alcohol or other CNS depressants with use of these agents.

ADVERSE REACTIONS:

CNS: Sedation, sleepiness, depression, lethargy, apathy, fatigue, disorientation, confusion, delirium, headache, slurred speech, stupor, coma, syncope, vertigo, nervousness, irritability.

Pulmonary: Respiratory disturbances (decreased tidal volume, respiratory rate, apnea).

Cardiovascular: Bradycardia, tachycardia, cardiovascular collapse, hypertension, hypotension, palpitations, edema.

GI: Constipation, diarrhea, dry mouth, nausea, anorexia, vomiting, increased salivation, gastritis.

Psychiatric: Behavior problems, hysteria, psychosis, suicidal attempt.

Other: Hiccoughs, fever, diaphoresis, paresthesias, muscular disturbances.

OVERDOSAGE:

Fatalities resulting from oral ingestion are not well documented. The oral agents rarely produce serious respiratory or circulatory depression. Overdose symptoms include ataxia, hypotonia, hypotension, and coma. IV administration of diazepam has resulted in hypotension and respiratory or cardiac arrest (1.7% incidence).

Treatment consists of inducing vomiting and monitoring respiration, pulse, and blood pressure. Maintain an adequate airway at all times. With normal kidney function, induce forced diuresis. In critical situations hemodialysis may be necessary. An agent, flumazenal, which has the ability to reverse the depressant effects of the benzodiazepines, is currently undergoing investigation (tentative trade name: Reversol). Table 16.2 lists some of the more commonly used benzodiazepines and related compounds.

NARCOTIC ANALGESICS

MECHANISM OF ACTION AND INDICATIONS FOR USE:

Narcotic analgesics comprise the opium alkaloids and their related derivatives. Specific receptor sites located throughout the CNS have been identified as opioid binding sites. Five categories of opioid receptors exist, with three categories being major action sites for narcotic analgesics. Of major concern to the practitioner are the mu (μ) receptors that enhance morphine-like analgesia at the supraspinal level, resulting in euphoria, respiratory depression, and physical depression. Morphine is a direct and continuous respiratory depressant that primarily suppresses the medullary respiratory center's response to increases in P_{CO_2}.

Narcotic analgesics are indicated for use to relieve moderate to severe pain

Table 16.2.
Common Benzodiazepines and Related Compounds

Benzodiazepine	Dose		Peak Plasma Level	Onset of Action
	Oral	IV		
	mg/day		*hr*	*min*
Long-acting				
Chlordiazepoxide (Librium)	15–100	25–50 mg tid, qid	1–4	PO: 30–60 IM: 15–30 IV: 3–30
Diazepam (Valium)	6–40	2–20 mg tid, qid	1–2	PO: 30–60 IM: 15–30 IV: rapid
Short-acting				
Lorazepam (Ativan)	2–6	2 mg up to 4 mg	1–6	PO: 30–60 IV: rapid
Midazolam HCl (Versed)	—	0.07 up to 0.6 mg/kg Range: 1 to 5 mg.	<1	IM: 15 IV: 3–5
Triazolan (Halcion)	0.25–0.5	—		PO: 30–60

(as with myocardial infarction), as a preoperative medication, as an adjunct during anesthesia, in patients with acute pulmonary edema due to left-sided heart failure, and for management and sedation of intubated patients. Some of these agents are also used for their antitussive effects (see also Chapter 7) and their antidiarrheal effects.

CONTRAINDICATIONS:

Hypersensitivity to narcotics, diarrhea caused by poisoning, premature infants, and during labor and delivery of premature infants.

PRECAUTIONS:

1. With repeated use tolerance, psychological dependence, and physical dependence may occur.
2. Use with extreme caution in patients with head injury and in patients with increased intracranial pressure. Along with the respiratory depressant effects, these agents have the ability to increase cerebrospinal fluid pressure.
3. Use with extreme caution in patients with asthma and in patients with other pulmonary disease owing to the agent's ability to severely diminish

respiratory drive, increase airway resistance, and suppress the cough mechanism.
4. Use with caution in the elderly, in debilitated patients, and in children.
5. Do not use concurrently with alcohol or other CNS depressants.

ADVERSE REACTIONS:

Major hazards: Respiratory depression, apnea, circulatory depression, respiratory arrest, shock, cardiac arrest.

Most frequent: Lightheadedness, dizziness, sedation, nausea, vomiting, sweating.

CNS: Euphoria, dysphoria, delirium, insomnia, agitation, anxiety, fear, hallucinations, disorientation, lethargy, coma, mood changes, headache, tremor, convulsions.

Cardiovascular: Tachycardia, bradycardia, hypotension, hypertension, palpitations, arrhythmias, syncope, peripheral circulatory collapse, facial flushing.

Table 16.3.
The Narcotics

	Dosage[a]				
Narcotic	IV	IM	Onset[b]	Peak[b]	Duration[b]
	mg	*mg*	*min*	*hr*	*hr*
Natural alkaloids of opium					
Morphine[c]	2–10	5–10	15–60	0.5–1	3–7
Codeine[c]	30–60	60–120	15–30	0.5–1	4–6
Semisynthetic derivatives					
Hydromorphone[c] (Dilaudid)	0.5–1	2	15–30	0.5–1	4–5
Oxymorphone (Numorphan)	0.5	1	5–10	0.5–1	3–6
Synthetic derivatives					
Fentanyl (Sublimaze)	0.05–0.1	0.1	7–8	—	1–2
Meperidine (Demerol)	25–100	50–100	10–45	0.5–1	2–4
Methadone (Dolophine)	2–5	2–10	30–60	0.5–1	4–6

[a]Dosage intervals: every 2 to 4 hours. Dosage range given is for a 70-kg adult.
[b]IM administration values.
[c]Strong antitussive effects.

Pulmonary: Respiratory depression, apnea, respiratory arrest, bronchospasm.
GI: Dry mouth, anorexia, constipation.

OVERDOSAGE:

Symptoms of severe overdosage occurring by IV injection include apnea, circulatory collapse, convulsions, cardiopulmonary arrest, and death. Complications of overdose include hypotension, bradycardia, hypothermia, pulmonary edema, pneumonia, and shock.

Treatment consists of maintaining an adequate airway with intubation and assisted respiration if necessary. Naloxone (Narcan, a narcotic antagonist) is the preferred drug to administer for reversal of narcotic overdose symptoms. The narcotics are listed in Table 16.3.

Additional narcotic analgesics include:

Sufentanil (Sufenta), Alfentanil (Alfenta)—given as primary anesthetic agents during cardiovascular surgery or neurosurgical procedures. Usually administered with 100% oxygen.

Orally administered narcotics:

Levorphanol (Levo-Dromoran); 2 mg preoperatively.
Oxycodone (Roxicodone); 5 mg every 6 hours.
Propoxyphene (Darvon); 65 mg every 4 hours.

MISCELLANEOUS RESPIRATORY DEPRESSANTS

Other drugs that may depress respiration if ingested in sufficiently high quantities (overdose) include formulations containing paraldehyde (Paral), chloral hydrate (Noctec), glutethimide (Doriden), propiomazine (Largon), Acetylcarbromal (Paxarel), methyprylon (Noludar), ethchlorvynol (Placidyl), and ethinamate (Valmid). Many of these are sleep-inducing preparations that are relatively safe if administered within the normal dosage range.

The antipsychotic drugs may also induce respiratory depression, cardiovascular collapse, coma, or cardiac arrest if administered in excessive quantities. These agents include the neuroleptics (such as Haldol, Thorazine, Compazene, Phenergan), the tricyclic antidepressants (such as Asendin, Surmontil, Sinequan), and the tetracyclic antidepressants (monoamine oxidase inhibitors, Ludiomil, Desyrel).

17 Respiratory Stimulants

The most commonly used drugs that cause central nervous system (CNS) stimulation and activation are the analeptics. At therapeutic doses, analeptic drugs exert their influence directly on the reticular activating center and on the vital centers located in the medulla. Another class of drugs that have CNS stimulating abilities is the narcotic antagonists. Also of interest as a respiratory stimulant is the hormone medroxyprogesterone acetate (MPA). For information concerning theophylline as a respiratory stimulant, refer to Chapter 12. Caffeine may also be considered as a stimulant; however, the large doses that are needed to stimulate respiration can also precipitate convulsions. Therefore, caffeine is generally not recommended to be administered as a respiratory stimulant.

Analeptic Agents

MECHANISM OF ACTION AND INDICATIONS FOR USE:

The major analeptic agent currently in use is doxapram. The older analeptics (pentylenetetrazol, picrotoxin, nikethamide) are not widely used anymore owing to their narrow margin of safety between the stimulating dose and the convulsant dose.

Doxapram is a powerful respiratory stimulant that elicits widespread CNS activation. In particular, doxapram enhances the rate and depth of respiration by directly activating the medullary respiratory center, as well as indirectly stimulating the aortic and carotid peripheral chemoreceptors. The degree of stimulation is directly dose related, and the duration of stimulation is seldom more than 5 or 10 minutes. Doxapram is currently the preferred drug of choice when an analeptic is indicated owing to its safety and efficacy as a respiratory stimulant.

Analeptics are indicated for use to stimulate respiration in postanesthetic patients, in drug-induced CNS depression, and in COPD patients associated with acute hypercapnia (only used as a temporary measure and not generally used concurrently with mechanical ventilation of these patients). These agents are also used in patients with congenital central hypoventilation syndrome, in patients with obesity-hypoventilation syndrome, and in neonates who exhibit respiratory depression, hypercapnia, and hypoventilation syndrome. Analeptics have also been used in neonatal apnea refractory to xanthine therapy.

CONTRAINDICATIONS:

Doxapram: Epilepsy, convulsive states, severe hypertension, cerebrovascular accidents, head injury, respiratory insufficiency due to pneumothorax, airway obstruction, dyspnea, asthma, pulmonary fibrosis.

PRECAUTIONS:

1. Administer cautiously with sympathomimetic amines; additive pressor effects may result.
2. Ensure patent airway and oxygenation prior to use.
3. Not to be used in conjunction with mechanical ventilation.
4. Safety and efficacy for use in children have not been established.
5. Use with extreme caution in patients with COPD due to possible arrhythmias secondary to hypoxia.
6. Use seizure precautions after the administration of these drugs.

ADVERSE REACTIONS:

CNS: Convulsions, headache, apprehension, dizziness, hyperactivity.

Pulmonary: Cough, dyspnea, tachypnea, laryngospasm, bronchospasm, rebound hypoventilation.

Cardiovascular: Arrhythmias, abnormal ECG, chest pain, flushing, tightness in chest.

GI: Nausea, vomiting, diarrhea.

OVERDOSAGE:

Respiratory alkalosis and hypocapnia with tetany and apnea. Excessive CNS stimulation may result in convulsions.

Treatment consists of supportive care. There is no specific antidote for overdosage of these agents; however, may have IV barbiturates, oxygen, and resuscitative equipment available.

DOSAGE:

Doxapram: Single intravenous bolus of 0.5 to 1 mg/kg in divided doses given at 5-minute intervals. Do not exceed 2 mg/kg. Doxapram is available in 20 mg/ml IV injection form and has a duration of activity of 3 to 4 minutes.

NARCOTIC ANTAGONISTS

MECHANISM OF ACTION AND INDICATIONS FOR USE:

Narcotic antagonists reverse narcotic-induced respiratory depression by competitively binding to the opioid receptor sites. Naloxone, in the absence of narcotics, does not produce any pharmacologic activity except for a slight drowsiness. Levallorphan, when used alone, may cause slight respiratory depression. These agents are not effective in reversing respiratory depression caused by nonnarcotic drugs, barbiturates, or anesthetics.

CONTRAINDICATIONS:

Hypersensitivity to these drugs. Acute liver disease, hepatitis.

PRECAUTIONS:

1. Maintain supportive therapy such as a patent airway and assisted respirations when indicated.
2. Administer with caution in patients who are known to be physically dependent on narcotic drugs.
3. Safety and efficacy in children have not been established.

ADVERSE REACTIONS:

An abrupt reversal of narcotic-induced depression may cause nausea, vomiting, sweating, tachycardia, hypertension, and tremors.

OVERDOSAGE:

Treat symptomatically, having resuscitation equipment available.

The narcotic antagonists are listed in Table 17.1.

MEDROXYPROGESTERONE ACETATE (MPA)
AMEN, CURRETAB, DEPO-PROVERA, PROVERA

MECHANISM OF ACTION AND INDICATIONS FOR USE:

MPA has the ability to stimulate alveolar ventilation and enhance the ventilatory response to hypercapnia and hypoxia. It is essentially useful in stimulating respirations in patients with obstructive sleep apnea.

Table 17.1.
The Narcotic Antagonists

Antagonist	Dosage Form	Dose[a]	Onset	Duration
			min	*hr*
Naloxone (Narcan)	IV, IM, SC: 0.4, 1 mg/ml	0.4 to 2 mg initially, may repeat IV at 2–3 minute intervals[b]	<5	1–4
Levallorphan (Lorphan)	IV: 0.05, 1 mg/ml	0.4 to 1 mg initially, then 0.5 mg at 10–15 minute intervals. Not to exceed 3 mg[b]	1	2–5
Naltrexone[c] (Trexan)	PO: 50-mg tablets	50 mg per day	60	24–72

[a]Total dose varies with patient and the degree of respiratory depression.
[b]Dosage range given is for reversal of narcotic overdosage.
[c]Indicated only for the prevention of narcotic use in former narcotic addicts.

ADVERSE REACTIONS:

Most common: Nervousness, insomnia, dizziness, depression, nausea, headache, breast tenderness, menstrual irregularities. Prolonged therapy may cause impotency in males.

DOSAGE:

MPA: 20 mg 3 times daily sublingual.

Anti-Infective Agents 18

In this chapter, the broad range of anti-infective agents are subdivided into five major categories: 1) the antibacterial (antibiotic) agents, 2) the antimycobacterial agents, 3) the antifungal agents, 4) the antiviral agents, and 5) the anti-infective agents specific for *Pneumocystis carinii.* Due to the wide variety of anti-infective agents, the primary purpose of this chapter is to focus on the most commonly used anti-infective agents that are indicated for use in respiratory tract infections and those agents used for infections in the critically ill patient. Table 18.2 summarizes some of the various anti-infectives used for specific infections.

Classification of Anti-Infective Agents

Several methods are used to classify and group the antimicrobial agents, many of which are based on the agent's chemical structure or mechanism of action. The following summarizes some of the more common methods used to classify these agents:

CATEGORY I: Consists of the agents that have the ability to inhibit the synthesis of the bacterial cell wall or to activate certain enzymes that disrupt the bacterial cell wall. Agents within this group include the penicillins, cephalosporins, vancomycin, and the antifungal agents such as ketoconazole and miconazole.

CATEGORY II: Consists of the agents that act directly on the microbe's cell membrane, causing leakage of the intracellular components. Agents within this group include amphotericin B, nystatin, and the detergents polymyxin and colistimethate.

Table 18.1.
Some Important Dates in the History of Microbiology and Antibiotic Development

Year	Accomplishment
1546	Girolamo Fracastoro of Verona suggested that a mysterious contagion could be passed from person to person through the air or by objects touched by people. Little attention was paid to these remarks. Disease, after all, was associated with magic and mysticism.
1676	Anton van Leeuwenhoek developed a crude lens system that magnified objects about 200 times. During the course of his work, he discovered tiny microbes, which he called "wee beasties." During a 50-year period, van Leeuwenhoek wrote over 200 letters describing the structure of thread-like fungi, several forms of bacteria and their movement, and the structure of the protozoa known today as the *paramecium* and *amoeba*. Even with these discoveries, microorganisms were just idle curiosities, nothing more. Van Leeuwenhoek invited no one to work with him, and showed no one the construction of his microscopes. By these actions, the development of microbiology was delayed almost 100 years until the instrumentation and the method of associating microbes with disease came together.
1859	Successful publication of Darwin's *On the Origin of Species* showed that the human body was susceptible to the laws of nature. It followed then that disease was a biological phenomenon apart from magic and mysticism and the involvement of microbes was a possibility that bore consideration.
1860 to 1885	Louis Pasteur disproved the theory of spontaneous generation, discovered that fermentation is caused by living yeasts, discovered immunization techniques, and developed the rabies vaccine. Robert Koch isolated the tubercle and cholera bacilli, developed pure culture techniques for microorganisms, and presented the germ theory of disease (proved that bacteria could be isolated and shown to cause disease). Christian Gram discovered and developed the Gram stain technique.
1870 to 1914	The "Golden Age of Microbiology." Most agents of bacterial disease were identified and cultivated.
1908	Salvarsan (the first chemotherapeutic agent) was developed by Paul Ehrlich.
1928	Sir Alexander Fleming isolated and identified penicillin.
1935	Sulfanilamide was discovered and developed. Sulfanilamide quickly became the principal agent for the treatment of war-related infections.

Table 18.1—*Continued*

Year	Accomplishment
1945	Sir Alexander Fleming, Ernst Boris Chain, and Sir Howard W. Florey received the Nobel Prize for discovery and development of penicillin. The discovery of the chemotherapeutic effects of sulfanilamide led to a renewed interest in penicillin. Penicillin was reisolated and made available for war-related infections. Since the 1940s, penicillin has remained the most important of the antibiotics due to its low cost and the broad use of the thousands of penicillin derivatives.
1949	The first broad-spectrum antibiotic, chloramphenicol, was introduced.
1950s	The β-lactam nucleus of the penicillin molecule was identified and synthesized, thereby creating new penicillins.
1952	Selman Waksman received the Nobel Prize for the discovery and development of streptomycin. Erythromycin was also discovered and developed at this time and was later shown to be a valuable antibiotic during outbreaks of atypical pneumonia in the 1970s.
1953	Tetracycline, a broad-spectrum antibiotic, was discovered and developed.
1954	John F. Enders, Thomas H. Weller, and Frederick C. Robbins received the Nobel Prize for cultivation of the polio viruses.
1957	Amphotericin B, the drug of choice for serious systemic fungal infections, was introduced.
1958	Vancomycin, especially useful for severe staphylococcal diseases where penicillin allergy or resistance exists, was introduced.
1963	Ampicillin, a valuable agent against certain Gram-negative rods and organisms of gonorrhea and meningococcal meningitis, was introduced.
1964	Nalidixic acid, the prototype of the quinolone group of drugs, was synthesized by Lesher *et al.* (1962) and introduced into clinical use.
1966	Gentamicin, one of the most popular of the aminoglycosides, was introduced.
1970	Clindamycin, an alternative agent used where penicillin resistance is found, was discovered and developed.
1971	Rifampin, a semisynthetic drug prescribed for tuberculosis and leprosy, was introduced.
1972	Spectinomycin, similar to streptomycin, was developed and introduced.
1980s	The newer second generation (ciprofloxacin, norfloxacin) of the quinolone drugs were developed for clinical use. These second generation quinolones have an expanded antibacterial spectrum that is active against most Gram-negative bacteria.

Table 18.2.
Recommended Antimicrobial Therapy for Infections[a,b]

Infecting Organism	Disease	Antibiotic of Choice	Alternative Drugs
Streptococcus pneumoniae	Pneumonia Endocarditis	Penicillin G	G1 cephalosporin, erythromycin
Staphylococcus aureus	Pneumonia Bacteremia Endocarditis	Penicillin G, nafcillin, or oxacillin	Vancomycin, G1 cephalosporin[c]
Streptococcus pyogenes	Pharyngitis Pneumonia Bacteremia	Penicillin G, penicillin V	G1 cephalosporin,[c] erythromycin
Corynebacterium diphtheriae	Pneumonia Pharyngitis Laryngotracheitis	Penicillin G	Erythromycin, G1 cephalosporin,[c] rifampin
Escherichia coli, Proteus, or *Enterobacter*	Pneumonia	Cefazolin + gentamicin	Cefotaxime + amikacin
Pseudomonas aeruginosa	Pneumonia Bacteremia	Ticarcillin or piperacillin + tobramycin	Other β-lactum antibiotic + an aminoglycoside
Klebsiella pneumoniae	Pneumonia	Cefazolin + gentamicin	Trimethoprim-sulfamethoxazole
Haemophilus influenzae	Bronchitis Sinusitis	Amoxicillin or ampicillin	Cefactor
Haemophilus influenzae	Epiglottitis Pneumonia	Chloramphenicol, cefotaxime, or moxalactam	Cefamandole, cefuroxime, or ampicillin
Legionella pneumophila	Legionnaires' disease	Erythromycin	Erythromycin + rifampin
Mycobacterium tuberculosis	Pulmonary	Isoniazid + rifampin	Isoniazid + rifampin + ethambutol
Aspergillus, Candida	Pneumonia	Amphotericin B	Amphotericin B + 5-fluorocytosine
Pneumocystis carinii	Pneumonia	Trimethoprim-sulfamethoxazole	Pentamidine

[a]Adapted from Gilman AG, Goodman LS, Rall TW, Murad F: Goodman and Gilman's the pharmacological basis of therapeutics. 7th ed. New York: Macmillan, 1985; and Pratt W: The antimicrobial drugs. Oxford, United Kingdom: Oxford University Press, 1986.

[b]This table focuses primarily on respiratory infections and a few other selected serious infections.

[c]G1, G3,—first- or third-generation cephalosporin.

Table 18.2—*Continued*

Infecting Organism	Disease	Antibiotic of Choice	Alternative Drugs
Francisella tularensis, *Yersinia pestis*	Pneumonia	Streptomycin	Chloramphenicol
Serratia marcescens	Pneumonia	Cefotaxime, or cefoxitin + amikacin	Trimethoprim-sulfamethoxazole
Bacteroides fragilis	Lung abscess Empyema Bacteremia Endocarditis Brain abscess	Clindamycin, metronidazole	Cefoxitin, or moxalactam
Bacteroides species (oral, pharyngeal)	Lung abscess Brain abscess Sinusitis	Penicillin G, clindamycin	Metronidazole, cefotoxitin, or moxalactam
Acinetobacter	Various nosocomial infections	An amino-glycoside	G3 cephalosporin

CATEGORY III: Consists of the agents that disrupt the functions of the bacterial ribosomes, causing the inhibition of protein synthesis. Agents within this group include chloramphenicol, clindamycin, erythromycin, and the tetracyclines.

CATEGORY IV: Consists of the agents that bind to the 30 S ribosomal subunit, thereby disrupting protein synthesis. The aminoglycosides compose this group.

CATEGORY V: Consists of the agents that alter the synthesis and metabolism of nucleic acid. Agents within this group include rifampin, the quinolone nalidixic acid and its derivatives, and metronidazole.

CATEGORY VI: Consists of the agents that have the ability to inhibit certain metabolic processes that are fundamental to the microorganism. Agents within this group include trimethoprim and the sulfonamides.

CATEGORY VII: Consists of the agents that inhibit viral replication by binding to the viral enzymes necessary for DNA synthesis. Vidarabine and acyclovir compose this group.

STAINING TECHNIQUES

The most important and simplest diagnostic tools available to determine the microorganism responsible for an infection are the Gram stain technique and the acid-fast staining technique.

The Gram stain technique is a differential diagnostic tool that allows the technician to separate bacteria into two groups. A small amount of bacteria (from samples such as sputum, urinary sediment, cerebrospinal fluid, or purulent drainage from the site of infection) is placed on a glass slide and allowed to air-dry. Next, the slide is passed through a flame (heat-fixing), which bonds the cells to the slide and kills most of the organisms to prepare them for the staining technique.

After heat-fixing, the slide is stained with crystal violet dye for 1 minute, then with Gram's iodine solution for another minute. All bacteria on the slide are now blue-purple. Next, the slide is rinsed with a decolorizer (such as 95% alcohol). During this process some bacteria completely lose all color and become transparent (Gram-negative bacteria), while other bacteria retain the blue-purple color (Gram-positive bacteria).

The last step in the Gram stain technique involves safranin, a red dye. When safranin is applied to the slide the Gram-negative bacteria absorb the stain and turn red-orange. At the conclusion of the procedure all Gram-positive bacteria are blue-purple, while all Gram-negative bacteria are red-orange.

The acid-fast staining technique is a diagnostic tool that determines the presence of bacteria of the genus *Mycobacterium*. These bacteria are very difficult to stain by conventional methods because of the waxy cell wall structure. Heat must be applied to force the dye molecules through to the bacteria's cytoplasm. Once these organisms are stained they are not easily decolorized by acids (hence, they are acid-resistant, or acid-fast).

A sample of respiratory secretions is placed on a glass slide and allowed to air-dry, then the slide is heat-fixed. Next, a Ziehl-Neelsen's carbolfuchsin stain is applied to the slide as it is heated. During this process all the cells on the slide turn a bright red color. The smear is then rinsed with an acid alcohol decolorizer; all acid-fast bacteria retain the red color (confirming the presence of *Mycobacterium*), while all other bacteria lose color and become transparent. A positive acid-fast test aids the physician in the diagnosis of tuberculosis.

SPECIFIC ANTIBACTERIAL AGENTS

PENICILLINS

MECHANISM OF ACTION:

The penicillins are bactericidal antibiotics that effectively kill bacteria by interfering with the synthesis of the bacterial cell wall. Specifically, they interfere with the synthesis of dipeptidoglycan, which gives the cell wall its strength and stability. Without the cell wall, lysis of the bacterial cell membrane occurs, and death follows. Penicillins are most effective during the active bacterial replication of young microorganisms. Penicillins have little or no effect on mature, dormant bacteria or bacteria that lack cell walls.

An intact β-lactam ring accounts for the penicillin's biological bactericidal activity. The side chain of the penicillin structure primarily determines the antibacterial spectrum. Narrow-spectrum penicillins act primarily on Gram-positive organisms. Broad-spectrum penicillins are effective not only on Gram-positive organisms but also on many Gram-negative bacilli.

The emergence of resistant strains of bacilli, either through mutations of the orginal infectious agent or through the ability of the bacilli to release enzymes (e.g., penicillinase) that can destroy the antibacterial drug, is a factor necessary to consider when administering these drugs.

INDICATIONS FOR USE:

The penicillins have remained for more than 5 decades as the most popular class of antibiotics in nonallergic patients. Modifications of the basic penicillin structure not only enables an enhanced activity against most Gram-positive and Gram-negative organisms, but also enables certain penicillins (e.g., cloxacillin, dicloxacillin, methicillin, nafcillin, and oxacillin) to resist enzymes (penicillinases) that convert penicillin to inactive penicilloic acid. Figures 18.1 to 18.3 summarize the organisms that are generally susceptible to the penicillins.

			Penicillinase-resistant					Aminopenicillins				Extended spectrum				
Gram-positive organisms	Penicillin G	Penicillin V	Methicillin	Nafcillin	Oxacillin	Cloxacillin	Dicloxacillin	Ampicillin	Bacampicillin	Amoxicillin	Cyclacillin	Carbenicillin	Ticarcillin	Mezlocillin	Piperacillin	Azlocillin
Staphylococci	●[1]	●[1]	●	●	●	●	●	●[1]	●[1]	●[1]	●[1]	●[1]	●[1]		●[1]	
Staphylococcus aureus	●[1]	●[1]	●	●	●	●	●					●[1]	●[1]	●[1]	●[1]	●[1]
Streptococci	●	●	●		●			●	●							
Streptococcus pneumoniae	●	●	●	●	●			●	●	●	●	●	●	●	●	●
Beta-hemolytic streptococci	●	●	●	●				●	●	●	●	●	●	●	●	●
Streptococcus faecalis	●	●						●	●	●		●	●	●	●	●
Streptococcus viridans	●	●		●						●					●	
Corynebacterium diphtheriae	●	●														
Bacillus anthracis	●	●						●								
Listeria monocytogenes	●	●						●								●

[1] Nonpenicillinase-producing.

Figure 18.1. Gram-positive organisms that are susceptible to the penicillins. (© 1990 by Facts and Comparisons. Used with permission from *Drug Facts and Comparisons. 1990 ed.* St. Louis: Facts and Comparisons, a Division of the J. B. Lippincott Company.)

Gram-negative organisms			Penicillinase-resistant					Aminopenicillins				Extended spectrum				
	Penicillin G	Penicillin V	Methicillin	Nafcillin	Oxacillin	Cloxacillin	Dicloxacillin	Ampicillin	Bacampicillin	Amoxicillin	Cyclacillin	Carbenicillin	Ticarcillin	Mezlocillin	Piperacillin	Azlocillin
Escherichia coli	●							●	●	●	●[3]	●	●	●	●	●
Hemophilus influenzae								●	●	●	●	●	●	●	●[2]	●
Klebsiella species														●	●	●
Neisseria gonorrhoeae	●[1]	●						●	●	●		●	●	●	●	
Neisseria meningitidis	●							●							●	
Proteus mirabilis	●							●	●	●	●[3]	●	●	●	●	●
Salmonella species	●							●				●	●		●	●
Shigella species	●							●						●	●	●
Morganella morganii												●	●	●	●	●
Proteus vulgaris												●	●	●	●	●
Providencia species																
Providencia rettgeri												●	●	●	●	●
Providencia stuartii														●		●
Enterobacter species	●											●	●	●	●	●
Citrobacter species												●	●	●	●	●
Pseudomonas aeruginosa												●	●	●	●	●
Serratia species												●	●	●	●	
Acinetobacter species														●	●	●
Streptobacillus moniliformis	●	●														

[1] Nonpenicillinase-producing.
[2] Non-beta-lactamase-producing.
[3] Only in the urinary tract.

Figure 18.2. Gram-negative organisms that are susceptible to the penicillins. (© 1990 by Facts and Comparisons. Used with permission from *Drug Facts and Comparisons. 1990 ed.* St. Louis: Facts and Comparisons, a Division of the J. B. Lippincott Company.)

CONTRAINDICATIONS:

Hypersensitivity to penicillin.

PRECAUTIONS:

1. Use with caution in patients with asthma, hay fever, or urticaria (hypersensitivity reactions may occur).
2. Do not use oral penicillin to treat severe pneumonia, empyema, bacteremia, meningitis, pericarditis, or purulent or septic arthritis during the acute stage.
3. Use with caution in neonates owing to an incompletely developed renal system.
4. Therapy must be of sufficient duration (at least 10 days and up to 4 weeks for severe infections) to completely eradicate the organism; otherwise, endocarditis or rheumatic fever may develop.

Anaerobic organisms	Penicillin G	Penicillin V	Methicillin	Nafcillin	Oxacillin	Cloxacillin	Dicloxacillin	Ampicillin	Bacampicillin	Amoxicillin	Cyclacillin	Carbenicillin	Ticarcillin	Mezlocillin	Piperacillin	Azlocillin
			Penicillinase-resistant					Aminopenicillins				Extended spectrum				
Clostridium species	●	●						●				●	●	●	●	●
Peptococcus species	●	●										●	●	●	●	●
Peptostreptococcus species	●	●										●	●	●	●	●
Bacteroides species	●[1]											●	●	●	●	●
Fusobacterium species	●											●	●	●	●	●
Eubacterium species	●												●	●	●	●
Treponema pallidum	●	●														
Actinomyces bovis	●	●														
Veillonella species													●	●	●	●

[1] *B. fragilis* is resistant.

Figure 18.3. Anaerobic organisms that are susceptible to the penicillins. (© 1990 by Facts and Comparisons. Used with permission from *Drug Facts and Comparisons. 1990 ed.* St. Louis: Facts and Comparisons, a Division of the J. B. Lippincott Company.)

5. Superinfection (secondary infection) may occur with the use of antibiotics due to bacterial or fungal overgrowth of nonsusceptible organisms.
6. Avoid concurrent use of other antibiotics (e.g., erythromycin, tetracycline). These agents may diminish the effectiveness of penicillin.

ADVERSE REACTIONS:

Allergic: Skin rashes, erythema, contact dermatitis, hives, wheezing, anaphylaxis, fever, eosinophilia, bronchospasm, laryngospasm, hypotension, vascular collapse.

CNS: Penicillin, carbenicillin, ampicillin, and ticarcillin have caused neurotoxicity when given in large IV doses and to patients with renal failure. Symptoms include lethargy, hallucinations, convulsions, seizures, and neuromuscular irritability.

GI: Diarrhea, abdominal cramps, nausea, vomiting, increased thirst.

Renal: Hematuria, pyuria, albuminuria, oliguria.

Miscellaneous: Superinfection, swelling of face and ankles, labored breathing, weakness, ecchymoses, hematomas.

OVERDOSAGE:

For severe allergic or anaphylactic reactions, administer epinephrine (0.3 to 0.5 ml of 1:1000 solution SC or IM, or 0.2 to 0.3 ml diluted with 10 ml saline given slowly by IV). Allergic reactions are more likely to occur in patients with asthma, hay fever, or urticaria. Severe or fatal potassium poisoning has occurred in patients receiving continuous IV therapy with potassium penicillin G in high dosage (10 to 100 million units/day).

Natural Penicillins

DOSAGE:

Penicillin G potassium	*For moderate to severe systemic infections:* ***PO:*** 1.6 to 3.2 million units/day, given every 6 hr in divided doses. ***IM, IV:*** 1.2 to 24 million units/day, given every 4 hr in divided doses. *Children:* ***PO:*** 25,000 to 100,000 units/kg/day, given every 6 hr in divided doses. ***IM, IV:*** 25,000 to 300,000 units/kg/day, given every 4 hr in divided doses.
Penicillin G procaine	*For moderate to severe systemic infections:* ***IM:*** 600,000 to 1.2 million units/day, given as single dose. *Children:* ***IM:*** 300,000 units/day, given as single dose.
Penicillin G sodium	*For moderate to severe systemic infections:* ***IM, IV:*** 1.2 to 24 million units/day, given every 4 hr in divided doses. *Children:* ***IM, IV:*** 25,000 to 300,000 units/kg/day, given every 4 hr in divided doses.
Penicillin V	*For moderate to severe systemic infections:* ***PO:*** 400,000 to 800,000 units (250 to 500 mg) every 6 hr. *Children:* ***PO:*** 25,000 to 90,000 units/kg/day (15 to 50 mg/kg), given every 6 to 8 hr in divided doses.

Aminopenicillins

DOSAGE:

Amoxicillin trihydrate Amoxil, Larotid, Polymox, Trimox	***PO:*** 750 mg to 1.5 g/day, given every 8 hr in divided doses. *Children:* ***PO:*** 20 to 40 mg/day, given every 8 hr in divided doses.
Ampicillin Amcap, Amcill, Ampicin, Polycillin, Supen, Totacillin, Probampacin	***PO:*** 1 to 4 g/day, given every 6 hr in divided doses. ***IM, IV:*** 2 to 12 g/day, given every 6 hr in divided doses. *Children:* ***PO:*** 50 to 100 mg/kg/day, given every 6 hr in divided doses.
Bacampicillin Penglobe, Spectrobid	***PO:*** 400 to 800 mg every 12 hr. *Children:* 25 to 50 mg/kg/day.

Cyclacillin Cyclapen-W	*PO:* 250 to 500 mg every 6 hr. *Children:* ***PO:*** 50 to 100 mg/kg/day, given every 6 hr in divided doses.

Penicillinase-resistant (Antistaphylococcal) Penicillins

DOSAGE:

Cloxacillin sodium Cloxapen, Tegopen	*PO:* 500 mg to 1 g every 4 to 6 hr. *Children:* ***PO:*** 50 to 100 mg/kg/day, given every 6 hr in divided doses.
Dicloxacillin sodium Dycill, Dynapen	***PO, IM:*** 250 mg to 1 g every 4 to 6 hr (maximum 4 g/day). *Children:* ***PO, IM:*** 25 to 50 mg/kg/day, given every 6 hr in divided doses.
Methicillin sodium Celbenin, Staphcillin	***IM, IV:*** 4 to 12 g/day, given every 4 to 6 hr in divided doses. *Children:* ***IM, IV:*** 100 to 200 mg/kg/day, given every 4 to 6 hr in divided doses.
Nafcillin sodium Nafcil, Unipen	***PO:*** 2 to 4 g/day, given every 6 hr in divided doses. ***IM, IV:*** 2 to 12 g/day, given every 4 to 6 hr in divided doses. *Children:* ***PO:*** 50 to 100 mg/kg/day, given every 4 to 6 hr in divided doses. ***IM, IV:*** 100 to 200 mg/kg/day, given every 4 to 6 hr in divided doses.
Oxacillin sodium Bactocill, Prostaphlin	***PO:*** 2 to 4 g/day, given every 6 hr in divided doses. ***IM, IV:*** 2 to 12 g/day, given every 4 to 6 hr in divided doses. *Children:* ***PO:*** 50 to 100 mg/kg/day, given every 6 hr in divided doses. ***IM, IV:*** 100 to 200 mg/kg/day, given every 4 to 6 hr in divided doses.

Extended-Spectrum Penicillins

DOSAGE:

Azlocillin sodium Azlin	***IV:*** (slow injection over a 5-minute period) 2 to 4 g every 4 to 6 hr.
Carbenicillin disodium Geopen	***IV:*** 30 to 40 g/day, given every 4 to 6 hr in divided doses. *Children:* ***IV:*** 300 to 500 mg/kg/day, given every 4 to 6 hr in divided doses.
Ticarcillin disodium Ticar	***IM, IV:*** 200 to 300 mg/kg/day, given every 4 to 6 hr in divided doses (3 g every 4 to 6 hr—maximum 2 g/injection IM). *Children:* 200 to 300 mg/kg/day, given every 4 to 6 hr in divided doses.

Mexlocillin sodium Mezlin	*IV:* 3 g every 4 hr (18 g/day) or 4 g every 6 hr (16 g/day).
Piperacillin sodium Pipracil	*IV:* 8 to 18 g/day, given every 6 to 8 hr in divided doses (dose depends upon severity of infection).

CEPHALOSPORINS AND CEPHAMYCINS

MECHANISM OF ACTION:

Cephalosporins are structurally and pharmacologically similar to the penicillins. These agents are the semisynthetic derivatives of *Cephalosporium acremonium.* Cephamycins are included due to their similarity to the cephalosporins. Cephalosporins inhibit the synthesis of the bacterial cell wall by interfering with mucopeptide biosynthesis, the final step in the formation of the cell wall. The unstable bacterial cell membrane disintegrates and the microorganism dies. Cephalosporins are more effective against rapidly growing microbes forming cell walls than on mature, dormant bacteria or those that lack cell walls.

INDICATIONS FOR USE:

The cephalosporins and cephamycins are indicated for use in a variety of mild to severe infections due to both Gram-positive and Gram-negative bacteria. These agents are subclassified into first, second, or third generation according to their broad or narrow antibacterial spectrum. The first-generation cephalosporins have a narrower antibacterial spectrum compared to the other generations of cephalosporins and are primarily effective against Gram-positive organisms, although they do exhibit some biological activity against a few Gram-negative species. The second-generation cephalosporins exhibit more activity against Gram-negative and some anaerobic bacteria than the first-generation cephalosporins. The third-generation cephalosporins have a broader antibacterial spectrum against aerobic Gram-negative bacilli, resistant organisms, and some anaerobic organisms than the first- and second-generation cephalosporins; however, the third-generation cephalosporins may be less effective against Gram-positive bacteria than first-generation cephalosporins. Figure 18.4 summarizes the organisms that are generally susceptible to the cephalosporins.

CONTRAINDICATIONS:

Hypersensitivity to these agents.

Organisms			
Staphylococci			
Streptococcus pneumoniae			
Beta-hemolytic streptococci	FIRST-		
Escherichia coli	GENERATION		
Hemophilus influenzae	CEPHALOSPORINS		
Klebsiella species			
Proteus mirabilis			
Streptococcus pyogenes			
Morganella morganii		SECOND-	
Providencia rettgeri		GENERATION	
Enterobacter species		CEPHALOSPORINS	
Clostridium species			
Peptococcus species			
Peptostreptococcus species			THIRD-
Fusobacterium species			GENERATION
Proteus vulgaris			CEPHALOSPORINS
Providencia species			
Neisseria gonorrhoeae			
Bacteroides species			
Neisseria meningitidis			
Salmonella species*			
Shigella species*			
Eubacterium species*			
*Clostridium difficile**			
Citrobacter species			
Serratia species			
*Salmonella typhi**			
Bacteroides fragilis			
Pseudomonas aeruginosa			
Acinetobacter species			

* Demonstrated in vitro activity.
Organisms may not exhibit susceptibility to each cephalosporin in a particular generation.

Figure 18.4. Summary of the organisms that are generally susceptible to the cephalosporins.

PRECAUTIONS:

1. Use with caution in patients with impaired renal or hepatic function owing to cephalosporin elimination by the kidneys. In most cases, the dosage must be adjusted according to the degree of renal impairment.
2. Use of these antibiotics may result in bacterial or fungal superinfection.

3. Avoid concurrent administration with other bacteriostatic agents; they may diminish the effectiveness of cephalosporins.

ADVERSE REACTIONS:

Most Common: Hypersensitivity and unwanted GI activity. Hypersensitivity is noted in patients with a history of asthma, allergy, hay fever, or urticaria. Hypersensitivity reactions range from mild to life threatening and include urticaria, rashes, pruritus, fever, chills, erythema, angioedema, and anaphylaxis.

GI: Nausea, vomiting, diarrhea, abdominal cramps, dyspepsia, heartburn.

CNS: Headache, dizziness, lethargy, paresthesia, seizures.

Miscellaneous: Hypotension, fever, dyspnea, interstitial pneumonitis.

First-Generation Cephalosporins

USES: Respiratory tract infections caused by *Streptococcus pneumoniae, Klebsiella* species, staphylococci, Group A β-hemolytic streptococci, *Haemophilus influenzae, Staphylococcus aureus.* Meningitis caused by *S. pneumoniae,* Group A β-hemolytic streptococci and staphylococci. Septicemia, endocarditis caused by *S. pneumoniae,* staphylococci, *Streptococcus viridans, Escherichia coli, Proteus mirabilis, Klebsiella* species, Group A β-hemolytic streptococci. Genitourinary infections caused by *E. coli, P. mirabilis, Klebsiella* species. Bone and joint infections caused by staphylococci, *S. aureus.* Skin and soft tissue infections caused by staphylococci, *E. coli, P. mirabilis, Klebsiella* species, Group A β-hemolytic streptococci.

DOSAGE:

Cefadroxil monohydrate Duricef, Ultracef	***PO:*** 1 to 2 g/day in a single dose or 2 divided doses. *Children:* 30 mg/kg/day. For pharyngitis and tonsillitis: 500 mg q 12 hr for 10 days.
Cefazolin sodium Ancef, Kefzol	***IM, IV:*** 250 to 500 mg q 8 hr up to 1 g q 6 hr for severe infections. Life-threatening infections (septicemia, endocarditis): up to 8 g daily given by IV. *Children:* 25 to 50 mg/kg/day, not to exceed 100 mg/kg/day.
Cephalexin monohydrate Keflex, Keftab, Keflet	***PO:*** 1 to 4 g/day in divided doses. Usual dose: 250 mg q 6 hr. *Children:* ***PO:*** 25 to 50 mg/kg/day; for severe infections, may double the dose.
Cephalothin sodium Keflin, Seffin	***IV:*** 500 mg to 1 g every 4 to 6 hr, or 4 to 12 g daily in divided doses (reserve higher doses for life-threatening conditions). *Children:* ***IV:*** 80 to 160 mg/kg/day.

Cephapirin sodium Cefadyl	*IM, IV:* 500 mg to 1 g q 4 to 6 hr, up to 12 g daily. *Children:* 40 to 80 mg/kg in 4 equally divided doses.
Cephradine Anspor, Velosef	***PO:*** 250 mg q 6 hr or 500 mg q 12 hr. ***IV:*** up to 8 g daily. *Children:* ***PO:*** 25 to 50 mg/kg/day. Not to exceed 4 g total daily dose. ***IM, IV:*** 2 to 4 g daily.

Second-Generation Cephalosporins

USES: Same antibacterial spectrum as first generation cephalosporins, in addition to lower respiratory tract infections, including pneumonia caused by *S. pneumoniae, H. influenzae,* and *S. pyogenes.* Also, upper respiratory tract infections caused by *S. pyogenes,* peritonitis caused by *E. coli* and *Enterobacter* species, intra-abdominal infections caused by *E. coli, Klebsiella* species, some *Bacteroides* species, and *Clostridium* species.

DOSAGE:

Cefaclor Ceclor	***PO:*** 250 mg q 8 hr, up to a maximum of 4 g daily. *Children:* 20 to 40 mg/kg/day, up to 1 g per day.
Cefamandole naftate Mandol	***IM, IV:*** 500 mg to 1 g q 4 to 8 hr, up to 2 g q 4 hr for life threatening infections. *Children:* 50 to 100 mg/kg/day, up to 150 mg/kg/day (not to exceed maximum adult daily dose).
Cefoxitin sodium Mefoxin	***IM, IV:*** 1 g q 6 to 8 hr, up to 4 g per day. For serious infections: 6 to 8 g per day. For life threatening infections: 12 g per day. *Children:* 80 to 160 mg/kg/day.
Cefonicid sodium Monocid	***IM, IV:*** 0.5 to 2 g once daily.
Ceforanide Precef	***IM, IV:*** 0.5 to 1 g q 12 hr. *Children:* 20 to 40 mg/kg/day.

Third-Generation Cephalosporins

USES: These agents are generally less active against Gram-positive cocci than first- or second-generation cephalosporins. Third-generation cephalosporins are primarily indicated for infections caused by *Neisseria meningitidis, H. influenzae, Citrobacter, Enterobacter, E. coli, Klebsiella* species, *N. gonorrhoeae, Proteus, Morganella, Providencia, Serratia, Pseudomonas aeruginosa,* and *Bacteroides fragilis.*

DOSAGE:

Cefoperazone sodium Cefobid	*IM, IV:* 2 to 4 g/day, up to 16 g/day for severe infections.
Cefotaxime sodium Claforan	*IM, IV:* 1 g per day, up to 12 g for life-threatening infections. *Children:* 50 to 180 mg/kg/day. ***ADDITIONAL USES:*** CNS infections (meningitis and ventriculitis) caused by *N. meningitidis, H. influenzae, S. pneumoniae, Klebsiella pneumoniae* and *E. coli.*
Ceftizoxime sodium Cefizox	*IM, IV:* 1 or 2 g q 8 to 12 hr, up to 12 g per day for life-threatening infections. *Children:* 50 mg/kg q 6 to 8 hr, up to 200 mg/kg/day.
Ceftriaxone sodium Rocephin	*IM, IV:* 1 to 2 g once a day, not to exceed a total daily dose of 4 g. *Children:* 50 to 75 mg/kg/day, not to exceed 2 g per day. For meningitis: 100 mg/kg/day, not to exceed 4 g per day.
Cefotetan disodium Cefotan	*IM, IV:* 1 to 4 g daily, up to 6 g for life-threatening infections.
Ceftazidime Fortaz, Tazicef, Tazidime	*IM, IV:* 250 mg q 12 hr, up to 2 g q 8 hr for serious infections. *Children:* 30 to 50 mg/kg q 8 hr, up to 6 g/day.
Moxalactam disodium Moxam	*IM, IV:* 2 to 6 g daily, up to 12 g/day. *Children:* 50 mg/kg q 6 to 8 hr, up to 200 mg/kg/day (not to exceed the adult daily dose).

AMINOGLYCOSIDES

MECHANISM OF ACTION:

The aminoglycosides irreversibly bind to the bacterial intracellular ribosomal 30S subunit. This action causes the inhibition of protein synthesis and alteration of the genetic code. The ribosomal unit separates from messenger RNA; cell death follows.

INDICATIONS FOR USE:

The aminoglycosides are broad-spectrum antibiotics indicated for a variety of severe, complicated, Gram-negative infections caused by *Pseudomonas, E. coli, Proteus, Klebsiella* species, *Serratia* species, *Providencia* species, *Acinetobacter* species, and *Enterobacter* species. The aminoglycosides are used concomitantly with other anti-infective agents to combat certain Gram-positive microorganisms such as *Staphylococcus aureus*, *Streptococcus faecalis*, and certain other streptococcus species and staphylococcus species. These drugs are not indicated for use in trivial infections or in those infections that can be eliminated with less toxic antibacterial agents due to their ototoxic and nephrotoxic potential. Figure 18.5 gives a summary of the organisms generally susceptible to the aminoglycosides.

CONTRAINDICATIONS:

Hypersensitivity to aminoglycosides. These agents are not indicated for long-term therapy (except for streptomycin used for tuberculosis) due to the ototoxic and nephrotoxic hazards.

PRECAUTIONS:

1. Use with caution in patients with neuromuscular disorders; aminoglycosides may increase muscle weakness due to a potential curare-like effect at the neuromuscular junction.
2. If these agents are used concurrently with penicillins or cephalosporins, a synergistic effect may be noted.
3. Monitor patient for the occurrence of superinfection.
4. Use with caution in renal impaired patients and in neonates and premature infants. Aminoglycosides are excreted primarily through glomerular filtration.

ADVERSE REACTIONS:

CNS: Confusion, disorientation, depression, lethargy, respiratory depression, headache, fever, acute organic brain syndrome, nystagmus, visual disturbances.

GI: Nausea, vomiting, anorexia, stomatitis.

Nephrotoxic: Proteinuria, hematuria, granular casts, azotemia, oliguria, rising BUN.

Ototoxic: Tinnitus, dizziness, vertigo, roaring in the ears.

Neurotoxic: Numbness, skin tingling, tremor, muscle twitching, neuromuscular blockade.

Miscellaneous: Myocarditis, palpitations, hypotension, hypertension, pulmonary fibrosis, hyperkalemia.

OVERDOSAGE:

To reduce excess serum levels, hemodialysis may be necessary.

DOSAGE:

Amikacin sulfate	***IM, IV:*** 15 mg/kg/day, given q 8 to 12 hr in divided doses.
Amikin	*Newborns:* loading dose of 10 mg/kg, then 7.5 mg/kg q 12 hr.

Group	Microorganisms	NEOMYCIN	STREPTOMYCIN	KANAMYCIN	GENTAMICIN	TOBRAMYCIN	AMIKACIN	NETILMICIN
Gram-positive	*Mycobacterium tuberculosis*		●[1]					
Gram-positive	*Staphylococcus* species				●[2]	●	●[2]	●[2]
Gram-positive	*Staphylococcus aureus*			●[2]		●		
Gram-positive	*Staphylococcus epidermidis*			●				
Gram-positive	*Streptococcus* species		●[1]					
Gram-positive	*Streptococcus faecalis*		●[1]	●[1]	●[1]	●[1]		●[1]
Gram-negative	*Acinetobacter* species			●			●	●
Gram-negative	*Citrobacter* species				●	●	●	●
Gram-negative	*Enterobacter* species				●	●	●	●
Gram-negative	*Enterobacter aerogenes*	●	●	●				
Gram-negative	*Escherichia coli*	●	●	●	●	●	●	●
Gram-negative	*Hemophilus influenzae*		●[1]	●				
Gram-negative	*Hemophilus ducreyi*		●					
Gram-negative	*Klebsiella* species	●	●[1]	●	●	●	●	●
Gram-negative	*Morganella morganii*					●		
Gram-negative	*Neisseria* species							●
Gram-negative	*Neisseria gonorrhoeae*			●				
Gram-negative	*Proteus* species	●	●	●[3]	●[3]	●[3]	●[3]	●
Gram-negative	*Proteus mirabilis*					●		●
Gram-negative	*Proteus vulgaris*	●				●		
Gram-negative	*Providencia* species					●	●	
Gram-negative	*Providencia rettgeri*					●	●	
Gram-negative	*Pseudomonas aeruginosa*	●			●[1]	●	●	●
Gram-negative	*Salmonella* species			●	●			●
Gram-negative	*Serratia* species			●	●	●	●	●
Gram-negative	*Shigella* species			●	●			●
Gram-negative	*Yersinia pestis*		●					

[1] Usually used concomitantly with other anti-infective agents.

[2] Penicillinase-producing and nonpenicillinase-producing.

[3] Indole-positive and indole-negative.

Figure 18.5. Organisms that are generally susceptible to the aminoglycosides. (© 1990 by Facts and Comparisons. Used with permission from *Drug Facts and Comparisons. 1990 ed.* St. Louis: Facts and Comparisons, a Division of the J. B. Lippincott Company.)

Gentamicin sulfate Garamycin	*IM, IV:* 3 to 5 mg/kg/day, given q 6 to 8 hr in divided doses. *Children:* 6 to 7.5 mg/kg/day (2 to 2.5 mg/kg q 8 hr). *Infants and neonates:* 2.5 mg/kg q 8 hr.
Kanamycin sulfate Kantrex, Klebcil	*IM, IV:* 15 mg/kg/day, up to 1.5 g per day, given q 8 to 12 hr in divided doses. ***PO:*** For hepatic coma: 8 to 12 g daily. Intestinal bacteria suppression preoperatively: 1 g q hr for 4 hr, then 1 g q 6 hr for 36 to 72 hr. ***Inhalation:*** 250 mg in saline nebulized bid or qid. *ADDITIONAL USES:* Primarily used orally for a number of aerobic bacteria in the GI tract preoperatively. This agent has also been used as an aerosol for respiratory tract infections.
Netilmicin sulfate	*IM, IV:* 4 to 6.5 mg/kg/day, given q 8 to 12 hr in divided doses. *Children:* 5.5 to 8 mg/kg/day. *ADDITIONAL USES:* Netilmicin has been effective in the treatment of serious infections caused by some organisms resistant to other aminoglycosides. Also, in combination with carbenicillin or ticarcillin for the treatment of life-threatening infections caused by *Pseudomonas aeruginosa.*
Streptomycin sulfate	*IM:* 1 to 2 g/day, given q 12 hr in divided doses. *Children:* 20 mg/kg/day. For tuberculosis: 1 g daily in combination with an antituberculous drug. *Children:* 20 to 40 mg/kg/day. For tularemia: 1 to 2 g daily. For plague: 2 to 4 g daily. Bacterial endocarditis: 1 g twice daily for one week, then 0.5 g twice daily for the second week; use in conjunction with penicillin. *ADDITIONAL USES:* Used in combination with antituberculous drugs to combat *Mycobacterium tuberculosis.* Also effective against a variety of serious infections in which less hazardous therapeutic agents are ineffective or contraindicated.
Tobramycin sulfate	*IM, IV:* 3 to 5 mg/kg/day, given q 6 to 8 hr in divided doses. *Neonates:* up to 4 mg/kg/day.

ERYTHROMYCIN

MECHANISM OF ACTION:

Erythromycin binds to the bacterial ribosomal 50S subunit, thereby suppressing protein synthesis and the transmission of genetic information. Erythromycin is effective against rapidly growing, reproducing microorganisms. The bacterial activity of erythromycin may be bactericidal or bacteriostatic depending on susceptible organisms and drug concentration.

INDICATIONS FOR USE:

Erythromycin is the drug of choice for respiratory infections caused by *Mycoplasma pneumoniae,* for Legionnaire's disease caused by *Legionella pneumophila,* for upper respiratory tract infections (otitis media) caused by *H. influenzae* when used in conjunction with sulfonamides. Also, erythromycin is effective against *Corynebacterium diphtheriae, Corynebacterium minutissimum,* and *Bordetella pertussis.* Erythromycin is also used as an alternative drug when penicillin or tetracycline is contraindicated or not tolerated, or when the patient exhibits hypersensitivity. Alternative uses include upper and lower respiratory infections (including pneumonia and bronchitis) caused by *Streptococcus pyogenes* and *S. pneumoniae,* skin and soft tissue infections caused by *S. pyogenes* and *S. aureus.* Also, pharyngitis, scarlet fever, cellulitis, and erysipelas caused by Group A *S. pyogenes.*

CONTRAINDICATIONS:

Hypersensitivity to erythromycin, preexisting liver disease (erythromycin estolate and ethylsuccinate).

PRECAUTIONS:

1. Use with extreme caution in patients with impaired hepatic function; these agents are principally excreted by the liver.
2. Monitor patient for superinfection.
3. Synergistic activity against *H. influenzae* has been noted with concomitant use with sufonamide.
4. Coadministered erythromycin with penicillin may decrease the effectiveness of penicillin; these drugs are rarely used together.

ADVERSE REACTIONS:

Allergic: Skin rashes, urticaria, eczema, anaphylaxis (rare).

GI: Oral dose-related side effects: abdominal cramps, anorexia, nausea, vomiting, diarrhea.

Miscellaneous: Superinfection.

DOSAGE (stated as erythromycin base):

Erythromycin base

E-mycin

Erythromycin estolate
Ilosone
Erythromycin ethylsuccinate
E.E.S., Erythrocin, Pediamycin, Wyamycin E, Eryped
Erythromycin gluceptate
Ilotycin
Erythromycin lactobionate
Erythrocin

PO: 250 mg q 6 hr, or 500 mg q 12 hr; for severe infections may give up to 4 grams daily. *Children:* 30 to 50 mg/kg/day; for severe infections may double the dose. ***IV:*** 15 to 20 mg/kg/day; for very severe infections may give up to 4 grams daily.

TETRACYCLINES

MECHANISM OF ACTION:

The tetracyclines are bacteriostatic antibiotics that inhibit protein synthesis by binding to the 30S ribosomal subunit.

INDICATIONS FOR USE:

Tetracyclines are used for a variety of Gram-positive, Gram-negative, aerobic, and anaerobic organisms and especially in infections caused by *Rickettsiae* (Rocky Mountain spotted fever, typhus fever, Q fever, rickettsialpox, tick fevers), *Chlamydia,* and *Mycoplasma pneumoniae.* Tetracyclines are not usually the drug of first choice for any staphylococcal infections or for infections that respond to penicillin; however, they are indicated for patients who are hypersensitive to penicillins and other antibiotics, or when bacteriologic testing demonstrates susceptibility of the organism to tetracycline.

CONTRAINDICATIONS:

Hypersensitivity to any of the tetracyclines.

PRECAUTIONS:

1. Tetracyclines are not generally used in children less than 8 years old, unless other drugs are contraindicated or are less effective. Tetracyclines cause

permanent discoloration in teeth during the formative tooth development period.

2. Use with caution in patients with renal impairment. Excessive systemic accumulation may occur.
3. Use of antibiotics may lead to bacterial or fungal overgrowth; secondary infection may occur.
4. Coadministered theophylline with tetracycline may increase the incidence of unwanted GI side effects.

ADVERSE REACTIONS:

CNS: Lightheadedness, dizziness, vertigo.

GI: Anorexia, nausea, vomiting, diarrhea, stomatitis, sore throat, dysphagia, hoarseness.

Renal: Increase in BUN.

Hepatic: Liver damage, pancreatitis.

Bones and Teeth: Permanent discoloration in teeth in children less than 8 years old. Temporary depressed bone growth in children and in fetuses.

DOSAGE:

Tetracycline HCl Achromycin V, Cyclinex, Tetra-C, Tetram, Cyclopar 500, Sumycin, Nor-Tet, Robitet	***PO:*** 250 to 500 mg q 6 hr. *Children >8 years:* 25 to 50 mg/kg/day in four divided doses. ***IM:*** 250 mg/day given in a single dose. *Children >8 years weighing <40 kg:* 15 to 25 mg/kg/day in divided doses at 8- to 12-hr intervals. ***IV:*** 250 to 500 mg bid at 12-hr intervals. *Children >8 years:* 20 to 30 mg/kg/day in divided doses at 8- to 12-hr intervals.
Oxytetracycline HCl Dilimycin, Oxlopar, Terramycin	***PO:*** 1 to 2 g/day, given in divided doses, do not exceed 500 mg q 6 hr. *Children >8 years:* 25 to 50 mg/kg/day in four divided doses. ***IM:*** 100 mg q 8 to 12 hr. *Children >8 years:* 15 to 25 mg/kg/day up to a maximum of 250 mg in a single daily dose. ***IV:*** 500 mg to 1 g daily in two doses. *Children >8 years:* 10 to 20 mg/kg/day in two divided doses.
Demeclocycline HCl Declomycin	***PO:*** 600 mg per day in two to four divided doses. *Children >8 years:* 6 to 12 mg/kg/day in two to four divided doses.
Methacycline HCl Rondomycin	***PO:*** 600 mg daily in two to four divided doses. *Children >8 years:* 10 mg/kg/day given in divided doses q 6 to 12 hr.

Doxycycline Vibramycin, Doxychel, Vivox, Doryx	***PO:*** 100 mg given at 12-hr intervals for two doses, followed by 100 mg given once daily. *Children >8 years and weighing less than 45 kg:* 4.4 mg/kg/day at 12-hr intervals for two doses, then 2.2 mg/kg once daily.
Minocycline HCl Minocin	***PO:*** Initially 200 mg, then 100 mg q 12 hr. *Children 8 to 12 years:* 4 mg/kg/day in divided doses q 12 hr. ***IV:*** *Adults:* same as PO. *Children >8 years:* Initially 4 mg/kg, then 2 mg/kg q 12 hr.

MISCELLANEOUS ANTIBACTERIAL AGENTS

CHLORAMPHENICOL
CHLOROMYCETIN

MECHANISM OF ACTION:
Chloramphenicol binds to the bacterial 50S ribosomal subunit, thereby inhibiting genetic transmission and protein synthesis.

INDICATIONS FOR USE:
This agent is the treatment of choice for typhoid fever caused by *Salmonella typhi* and serious infections caused by *Salmonella* (e.g., bacteremia), *Rickettsia* (when tetracyclines are contraindicated), and *Chlamydia*. Also, epiglottitis and cellulitis caused by *H. influenzae* that is resistant to ampicillin.

CONTRAINDICATIONS:
Hypersensitivity. Chloramphenicol is not to be used for trivial infections or as prophylaxis for bacterial infections. This agent is indicated for serious infections in which less dangerous drugs are ineffective or contraindicated.

PRECAUTIONS:
1. Use with caution in patients with impaired renal and hepatic functions.
2. Monitor patient for superinfection.

ADVERSE REACTIONS:
Most Serious: Blood dyscrasias (aplastic anemia, hypoplastic anemia, thrombocytopenia, and granulocytopenia).
CNS: Headache, depression, confusion, delirium.
GI: Nausea, vomiting, glossitis, stomatitis, diarrhea.

DOSAGE: ***PO:*** 50 to 100 mg/kg/day in divided doses every 6 or 8 hr. Higher doses are reserved for exceptional infections (e.g., meningitis, brain abscess).

IV: Administer as a 10% solution injected over at least 1 minute. Substitute oral dosage as soon as feasible.

CLINDAMYCIN
CLEOCIN HYDROCHLORIDE, CLEOCIN PHOSPHATE

MECHANISM OF ACTION:

Clindamycin has the ability to prevent bacterial protein synthesis by binding to the 50S subunit of bacterial ribosomes.

INDICATIONS FOR USE:

Clindamycin is effective against and indicated for serious respiratory tract infections (such as empyema, anaerobic pneumonitis, and lung abscess). Also, for serious skin and soft tissue infections. Clindamycin is effective against Gram-positive organisms such as *S. aureus, Staphylococcus epidermidis, Staphylococcus pyogenes, S. pneumoniae,* β-hemolytic streptococci, *S. viridans, C. diphtheriae,* and *Nocardia asteroides.* Clindamycin is also indicated for infections caused by anaerobic organisms such as *Fusobacterium, Bacteroides, Clostridium perfringens, Eubacterium, Actinomyces* species, *Peptococcus, Peptostreptococcus,* microaerophilic streptococci, *Clostridium tetani,* and *Veillonella.* For anaerobic infections, clindamycin is initially given parenterally, then may be followed by oral therapy.

CONTRAINDICATIONS:

Hypersensitivity. Clindamycin is not to be used for minor bacterial or viral infections owing to its serious adverse side effects.

PRECAUTIONS:

1. Use with caution in patients with history of asthma or allergies, owing to possible hypersensitivity reactions.
2. Use with extreme caution in patients with history of GI disease, especially colitis (clindamycin may cause severe or fatal colitis). Patients should be instructed to report diarrhea and not to treat such diarrhea himself or herself.
3. Renal, hepatic, and hematopoietic functions should be monitored during prolonged therapy.
4. Erythromycin should not be used concurrently with clindamycin; erythromycin may block clindamycin's ability to inhibit bacterial protein synthesis.
5. Appropriate measures should be taken if superinfection occurs.

6. Clindamycin may enhance the actions of neuromuscular blocking agents; use cautiously.
7. Each oral dose of clindamycin should be taken with a full glass of water to avoid esophageal irritation.

ADVERSE REACTIONS:

Cardiovascular: Hypotension, cardiopulmonary arrest (following too rapid IV administration—rare occurrence).
GI: Nausea, vomiting, diarrhea, pseudomembranous colitis, abdominal pain, esophagitis, anorexia.
Miscellaneous: Neutropenia, leukopenia, jaundice, skin rashes, urticaria.

DOSAGE: ***PO:*** 150 to 450 mg q 6 hr. ***IM, IV:*** 600 to 1200 mg/day up to 2.7 g/day (for more severe infections) in two to four divided doses. Life-threatening occurrences: up to 4.8 g/day given IV. *Children:* 8 to 25 mg/kg PO daily; or 15 to 40 mg/kg IM or IV given daily in three to four equal doses.

VANCOMYCIN HYDROCHLORIDE
VANCOCIN HYDROCHLORIDE

MECHANISM OF ACTION:

Vancomycin inhibits bacterial cell wall biosynthesis by binding to the cell walls of reproducing microorganisms. Through this action, vancomycin alters the cellular membrane permeability and RNA synthesis.

INDICATIONS FOR USE:

Vancomycin is indicated for serious life-threatening infections (including methicillin-resistant staphylococci) caused by Gram-positive cocci (*S. pyogenes, S. pneumoniae*) and is the most potent antibiotic available for infections caused by *S. aureus* and *S. epidermidis*. Vancomycin is also effective, alone or in combination with an aminoglycoside, for endocarditis caused by *S. viridans* or *Streptococcus bovis*.

CONTRAINDICATIONS:

Hypersensitivity. Due to this drug's serious adverse effects, vancomycin is reserved for potentially life-threatening infections that are not treatable with other less toxic antibiotics, including the penicillins and cephalosporins.

PRECAUTIONS:
1. Avoid rapid IV bolus administration; may cause serious hypotension, cardiac arrest.
2. Use cautiously in renal impaired patients owing to the drug's nephrotoxicity.
3. Use cautiously in patients with previous hearing loss owing to the drug's potential ototoxicity.
4. As with all antibiotics, monitor patient for superinfection.

ADVERSE REACTIONS:
Most Serious: Ototoxicity, nephrotoxicity.
Other: Nausea, urticaria, macular rashes, chills, eosinophilia, anaphylactic reactions.

DOSAGE: ***PO:*** 500 mg every 6 hours or 1 g every 12 hours. ***IV:*** Same dose as oral. *Children:* 40 mg/kg/day in 4 divided doses. Not to exceed 2 g per day. ***IV:*** Same dose as oral.

Quinolones

Most of the new quinolone derivatives are still investigational; however, the newer second-generation quinolones that are now available include ciprofloxacin and norfloxacin. Norfloxacin's primary indication is for the treatment of complicated and uncomplicated urinary tract infections; therefore this section focuses on ciprofloxacin, a bactericidal antibiotic useful for a variety of Gram-negative and Gram-positive organisms.

CIPROFLOXACIN HYDROCHLORIDE
CIPRO

MECHANISM OF ACTION:
Ciprofloxacin interferes with the enzyme DNA gyrase, which is needed for bacterial DNA synthesis. The increased bacterial susceptibility to this newer quinolone, as compared to nalidixic acid, may be related to its superior capability to penetrate the bacterial outer membrane.

INDICATIONS FOR USE:
This agent is especially useful for lower respiratory tract infections caused by *E. coli, K. pneumoniae, Enterobacter cloacae, P. mirabilis, P. aeruginosa, H. influenzae, Haemophilus parainfluenzae,* and *S. pneumoniae.* Also, infections

caused by *S. aureus* (including those that are methicillin susceptible and methicillin resistant), *S. pyogenes*, and *S. pneumoniae*.

CONTRAINDICATIONS:
Hypersensitivity. Also hypersensitivity to the older quinolones may contraindicate use.

PRECAUTIONS:
1. Additive effects may be noted when ciprofloxacin is used with other agents such as β-lactams or aminoglycosides.
2. Prolonged or repeated use may result in superinfection.
3. Ciprofloxacin is contraindicated in children due to the emergence of arthropathy in immature animals.
4. Avoid concurrent use of antacids with ciprofloxacin therapy. Antacids may inhibit the absorption of ciprofloxacin.
5. Concurrent use with theophylline may result in increased theophylline-related adverse reactions.
6. Ciprofloxacin may be taken with or without meals; however, the preferred time is 2 hours after a meal. Liberal use of fluids is recommended.
7. Observe caution when performing tasks that require alertness; ciprofloxacin may cause drowsiness and dizziness.

ADVERSE REACTIONS:
Most Frequent: Nausea, diarrhea, vomiting, abdominal discomfort, headache, restlessness, and rash.

DOSAGE: ***PO:*** Mild to moderate infections: 250 to 500 mg every 12 hours. Severe or complicated infections: up to 750 mg every 12 hours. For patients with impaired renal function, the recommended dose is ½ that of the usual dose; however, serum drug levels indicate the most reliable method for dosage adjustment.

Antimycobacterial Agents

MECHANISM OF ACTION:
Antituberculosis drugs interfere with cell wall synthesis in tubercle bacilli. These agents are categorized as first-line drugs (primary), second-line drugs

(secondary), and tertiary drugs. The second-line drugs and tertiary drugs are indicated for use only in combination with the first-line drugs in which drug resistant mycobacteria are present. Second-line and tertiary drugs are not as effective and are generally more toxic than first-line drugs.

INDICATIONS FOR USE:

These agents are indicated for all forms of tuberculosis and as preventive therapy. Many of these agents are used in combination with each other for effective control of tuberculosis. Examples are isoniazid 300 mg and rifampin 600 mg, both administered in single daily doses. Sputum conversion (failure of growth of *M. tuberculosis* in sputum cultures) usually occurs within 1 month. Other antituberculosis regimens include isoniazid-streptomycin-ethambutol given as initial therapy followed by isoniazid-ethambutol and continued for 18 to 24 months.

Recently, the American Thoracic Society and the Tuberculosis Control Division of the Centers for Disease Control have endorsed a 9-month regimen of isoniazid-rifampin as an alternative for adults who have had previously untreated, uncomplicated pulmonary tuberculosis.

CONTRAINDICATIONS:

Hypersensitivity. Patients with hepatic injury or acute liver disease (isoniazid).

PRECAUTIONS:

1. Monitor patient for signs of hepatitis. The risk of developing hepatitis increases with age and daily alcohol comsumption.
2. Use cautiously in patients with renal and liver impairments.

ADVERSE REACTIONS:

Serious toxic effects are usually dose related, with the most common effects affecting the nervous system and the liver.

Nervous System: Peripheral neuropathy (isoniazid, ethionamide). Other neurotoxic effects include convulsions, optic neuritis, memory impairment, and toxic psychosis.

CNS: Headache, drowsiness, confusion, inability to concentrate, possible hallucinations.

GI: Nausea, vomiting.

DOSAGE:

	Adult Daily Dose	Pediatric Daily Dose	Activity
	mg/kg	*mg/kg*	
PRIMARY DRUGS			
Isoniazid	5 to 10 (single dose)	10 to 20 max-500 mg/day	Bactericidal
Rifampin	10 (single dose)	10 to 20 max-600 mg/day	Bactericidal
SECONDARY DRUGS			
Ethambutol	15 to 25 (single dose)	15	Bacteriostatic
Pyrazinamide	20 to 35 (single dose)	20 to 30	Bactericidal
Streptomycin[a]	15 to 25 (single dose)	20 to 40	Bactericidal
TERTIARY DRUGS			
Capreomycin[a]	15 (single dose)	—	Bactericidal
Cycloserine	10 to 15 (four divided doses q 6 hr)	5 to 15	Bacteriostatic
Ethionamide	7 to 15 (four divided doses q 6 hr)	10 to 20 max-750 mg/day	Bacteriostatic
Kanamycin[a]	15 (single dose)	—	Bactericidal
P-aminosalicylic acid	200 (four divided doses q 6 hr)	200 to 420	Bacteriostatic

[a]IM route only; all other drugs are given orally.

ANTIFUNGAL AGENTS

Fungal infections are of three types:

1. Dermatophytic—Infections that involve the hair, skin, and nails. These infections are treated topically with preparations such as Desenex, Aftate, Halotex, Lotrimin, or Monistat-Derm, depending on the causative orga-

nism. Causative organisms include *Epidermophyton, Trichophyton,* and *Microsporum.*
2. Mucocutaneous—These infections include only candidiasis. Moist skin and mucous membranes are the areas infected. Causative organisms include *Candida albicans* (most common), *Candida tropicalis,* and *Candida parapsilosis.*
3. Systemic—These infections are classified as deep or subcutaneous. Organisms causing deep systemic mycoses generally enter the body through inhalation, then spread to other organs. Infections such as aspergillosis, blastomycosis, coccidioidomycosis, cryptococcosis, histoplasmosis, mucormycosis, and paracoccidioidomycosis are generally deep mycoses. Some subcutaneous mycoses include chromomycosis, mycetoma, and sporotrichosis. Subcutaneous infections usually enter the body through the skin, then spread to adjacent tissues.

This section concentrates on the more serious, potentially life-threatening systemic fungal infections and the anitfungal drugs used to treat these infections.

AMPHOTERICIN B
FUNGIZONE

MECHANISM OF ACTION:

Amphotericin B is a fungicidal antibiotic that has the ability to bind to the fungal cell membrane and alter the cellular permeability, thereby inhibiting growth and reproduction of the organism. Amphotericin B is selective in that it exerts its influence only on fungal cell membranes (due to the presence of sterol in the cellular membrane). Bacteria and viruses do not contain the component sterol in their cellular membranes; therefore, amphotericin B is ineffective against these organisms.

INDICATIONS FOR USE:

Amphotericin B is the drug of choice for systemic fungal infections and is specifically intended to treat blastomycosis, candidiasis, cryptococcosis, histoplasmosis, and paracoccidioidomycosis. Mucormycosis, aspergillosis, and sporotrichosis infections also respond to amphotericin B.

CONTRAINDICATIONS:

Hypersensitivity, unless the infection is life-threatening and responsive only to amphotericin B.

PRECAUTIONS:

1. Monitor patient for signs of renal damage, the most important toxic adverse effect of amphotericin B therapy.
2. Potentiation of effects is noted with coadministered digitalis and skeletal muscle relaxants.

ADVERSE REACTIONS:

Most Common: Fever, headache, chills, anorexia, muscle and joint pain, nausea, vomiting, diarrhea.

Renal: Hypokalemia, azotemia, hyposthenuria.

Pulmonary: Acute dyspnea, hypoxemia, interstitial infiltrates in neutropenic patients.

DOSAGE: *IV:* Individualized dosage depending on the severity of the disease: Do not exceed a total daily dose of 1.5 mg/kg. Several months of therapy is usually necessary.

FLUCYTOSINE
ANCOBON

MECHANISM OF ACTION:

The exact mode of action of flucytosine is unknown; however, it is metabolized to fluorouracil within the fungal cell and is known to produce synergistic activity when coadministered with amphotericin B.

INDICATIONS FOR USE:

For the treatment of serious infections (septicemia, endocarditis, meningitis, and pulmonary infections) caused by strains of *Candida* and *Cryptococcus.* Flucytosine is usually used in conjunction with amphotericin B due to the emergence of resistant strains of *Candida.*

CONTRAINDICATIONS:

Hypersensitivity.

PRECAUTIONS:

1. Monitor patients frequently for renal status; drug accumulation may occur in renally impaired patients.
2. Use cautiously in bone marrow depressed patients; this drug may potentiate bone marrow depression.
3. Although coadministration of amphotericin B is usually therapeutic, it also increases the incidence of toxicity.

ADVERSE REACTIONS:

Most Frequent: Nausea, vomiting, diarrhea, rash, anemia, leukopenia, thrombopenia.

Less Frequent: Confusion, hallucinations, headache, drowsiness, vertigo.

DOSAGE: ***PO:*** 50 to 150 mg/kg/day in divided doses given at 6-hr intervals. With amphotericin B (0.3 mg/kg/day): 150 mg/kg/day in four divided doses.

KETOCONAZOLE
NIZORAL

MECHANISM OF ACTION:

Ketoconazole is a recently developed antifungal agent that alters the fungal plasma membrane by interfering with the biosynthesis of ergosterol. This action causes the leakage of cellular components, promoting the death of the fungal cell.

INDICATIONS FOR USE:

Ketoconazole is indicated for and effective against both mucocutaneous and systemic fungal infections of candidiasis, chronic mucocutaneous candidiasis, oral thrush, candiduria, blastomycosis, coccidioidomycosis, histoplasmosis, chromomycosis, and paracoccidioidomycosis. High doses of ketoconazole have been effective against CNS fungal infections.

CONTRAINDICATIONS:

Hypersensitivity. Not to be used in the treatment of fungal meningitis owing to the poor penetration of the drug into the cerebral spinal fluid.

PRECAUTIONS:

1. Do not use this drug in direct conjunction with antacids, anticholinergics, or H_2 blockers. These agents may block the effect of ketoconazole due to their alkaline environment. Dissolution and absorption of the drug may be impaired.

ADVERSE REACTIONS:

CNS: Headache, dizziness, somnolence, photophobia.

GI: Nausea, vomiting, abdominal pain, diarrhea.

DOSAGE: ***PO:*** 200 mg given in a single daily dose, up to 400 mg daily for serious infections. *Children >2 years:* 3.3 to 6.6 mg/kg/day.

MICONAZOLE
MONISTAT IV

MECHANISM OF ACTION:
Miconazole is a broad-spectrum antifungal agent that alters the permeability of the fungal plasma membrane, thereby causing the leakage of cellular components.

INDICATIONS FOR USE:
Miconazole is effective in the treatment of severe fungal infections such as coccidioidomycosis, candidiasis, cryptococcosis, petriellidiosis, paracoccidioidomycosis, and chronic mucocutaneous candidiasis, Miconazole is not indicated in the treatment of trivial fungal diseases. Miconazole is an alternative drug to amphotericin B in patients with renal impairment or those who do not tolerate amphotericin B therapy.

CONTRAINDICATIONS:
Hypersensitivity.

PRECAUTIONS:
1. Administer drug by slow IV infusion; rapid infusion may cause transient tachycardia or arrhythmias.
2. Amphotericin B and miconazole have been noted to have antagonistic properties; that is, when these drugs are given concurrently, the effects produced are less than when they are given alone.

ADVERSE REACTIONS:
GI: Nausea, vomiting, diarrhea, anorexia.
Other: Fever, drowsiness, flushes, decrease in serum sodium levels.

DOSAGE: *IV injection, total daily dosage range (mg):*

For coccidioidomycosis:	1800 to 3600
For cryptococcosis:	1200 to 2400
For petriellidiosis:	600 to 3000
For candidiasis:	600 to 1800
For paracoccidioidomycosis:	200 to 1200

Children: 20 to 40 mg/kg/day. Not to exceed 15 mg/kg per infusion.
Duration of therapy ranges from 1 to >20 weeks.

ANTIVIRAL AGENTS

Classification of Viruses

Viruses are initially classified according to the viral genome (hereditary factors), which may contain either ribonucleic acid (RNA) or deoxyribonucleic acid (DNA), but never both. The following list includes some of the more common RNA and DNA viruses and the infectious diseases they cause.

RNA VIRUS	DISEASES
Coronaviridae	Coronaviruses (respiratory infections)
Orthomyxoviridae	Influenza viruses
Paramyxoviridae	Parainfluenza viruses (croup, pneumonia, bronchitis), measles virus, respiratory syncytial virus (bronchiolitis, pneumonia)
Picornaviridae	Polioviruses, coxsackieviruses, echoviruses (aseptic meningitis), rhinoviruses, hepatitis infections
Reoviridae	Rotaviruses (diarrhea), Colorado tick fever, respiratory infections
Retroviridae	Retroviruses (primary agent of acquired immune deficiency syndrome [AIDS], also known as the human immunodeficiency virus [HIV])
Rhabdoviridae	Rabies virus
Togaviridae	Encephalitis viruses (mosquito borne), yellow fever viruses, rubella virus

DNA VIRUS	DISEASES
Adenoviridae	Adenoviruses (acute respiratory diseases)
Herpesviridae	Herpes simplex types 1 and 2, varicella-zoster (chickenpox, shingles), cytomegalovirus, Epstein-Barr virus (mononucleosis)
Papovaviridae	Papilloma viruses (warts)
Poxviridae	Variola virus (smallpox)

SPECIFIC ANTIVIRAL DRUGS

AMANTADINE HYDROCHLORIDE
SYMMETREL

MECHANISM OF ACTION:

Amantadine acts to uncoat the RNA virus, thereby blocking the transfer of viral nucleic acid into the host cell.

INDICATIONS FOR USE:
Amantadine is specific for the prevention and treatment of respiratory tract infections caused by influenza A virus strains. Early immunization is the treatment of choice, especially for high-risk patients with underlying disease states.

CONTRAINDICATIONS:
Hypersensitivity.

PRECAUTIONS:
1. Use with caution in patients with liver disease, CHF, and renal impairment and in the elderly. Dosage may need to be reduced or adjusted.
2. CNS effects include blurred vision. Use with caution while driving or performing other similar tasks.
3. Monitor patient carefully if CNS stimulants are administered concurrently.

ADVERSE REACTIONS:
Most Frequent: CNS side effects including confusion, hallucinations, anxiety, insomnia, lightheadedness. Depression of mental alertness.
Less Frequent: Vomiting, headache, dyspnea, fatigue.

DOSAGE: ***PO:*** 200 mg as a single dose or 100 mg bid. *Children 9 to 12 years:* 100 mg bid. *Children 1 to 9 years:* 2 to 4 mg/lb/day, not to exceed 150 mg/day.

RIBAVIRIN
VIRAZOLE

MECHANISM OF ACTION:
Ribavirin is an antiviral agent with selective inhibitory activity against respiratory syncytial virus (RSV), influenza virus, and herpes simplex virus. The mechanism of action of ribavirin is unknown.

INDICATIONS FOR USE:
Ribavirin aerosol is indicated for infants and young children with *severe* lower respiratory tract infections caused by RSV. Ribavirin aerosol is not indicated for RSV infections not accompanied by severe lower respiratory tract infections; therefore the decision to treat patients with RSV infections is based upon the severity of the RSV infection. This drug should not be administered without documentation of RSV due to its serious adverse effects.

CONTRAINDICATIONS:
Pregnancy, known or suspected. Ribavirin has been found to be teratogenic.

PRECAUTIONS:

1. The presence of prematurity or existing cardiopulmonary disease in infants and young children may increase the severity of the RSV infection.
2. Ribavirin aerosol is generally not indicated for use in patients requiring assisted ventilation (not approved by the FDA). Precipitation of the drug may occur, hindering safe and effective ventilation.
3. Worsening of respiratory status with ribavirin use has been noted in infants and in adults with chronic obstructive lung disease.
4. Careful monitoring of respiratory and fluid status is required in patients with severe lower respiratory tract infections due to RSV.
5. Ribavirin administered by aerosol is absorbed systemically.
6. Aerosolized ribavirin may escape into the air around the patient, therefore both visitors and staff may be exposed to the drug. Due to the serious adverse reactions that ribavirin *may* cause to visitors and staff, as with other potentially hazardous drugs, pregnant women should avoid exposure to the drug.

ADVERSE REACTIONS:

Cardiovascular: Cardiac arrest, hypotension, digitalis toxicity.

Pulmonary: Deteriorating respiratory function, bacterial pneumonia, pneumothorax, apnea, ventilator dependence.

Pregnancy: Teratogenic effects.

Miscellaneous: Rash, conjunctivitis.

DOSAGE: Ribavirin aerosol may be administered only through a Small Particle Aerosol Generator (SPAG). Complete familiarity with this system is essential before use (refer to Viratek SPAG-2 Operator's Manual for operating instructions). Treatment is usually effective if initiated within 3 days after the onset of RSV lower respiratory tract infection and is carried out for 12 to 18 hours per day for 3 to 7 days. Use of the SPAG-2 aerosol generator requires an infant oxygen hood, face mask, or oxygen tent.

Ribavirin aerosol is supplied in 100-ml vials as 6 grams of lyophilized drug. To administer, solubilize the drug with sterile USP water for injection or inhalation in the 100-ml vial. Transfer the solution to the 500-ml wide-mouthed Erlenmeyer flask (SPAG-2 reservoir). Add sterile USP water for injection or inhalation to obtain a total volume of 300 ml. The final concentration is 20 mg/ml. **Warning:** The sterile USP water for injection or inhalation should not have any antimicrobial agent or other substance added. Discard used solution every 24 hours and before adding newly reconstituted solution.

ZIDOVUDINE (AZT)
RETROVIR

MECHANISM OF ACTION:
Zidovudine inhibits viral replication of some retroviruses, including human immunodeficiency virus (HIV), by interfering with the HIV viral RNA-dependent DNA polymerase (reverse transcriptase).

INDICATIONS FOR USE:
The Food and Drug Administration has approved zidovudine to treat certain adult patients with symptomatic HIV infections (AIDS and AIDS-related complex [ARC]). However, this drug does not cure AIDS.

CONTRAINDICATIONS:
Patients who exhibit life-threatening allergic reactions to any of zidovudine's components.

PRECAUTIONS:
1. Coadministered acetaminophen may increase the toxicity of zidovudine.
2. Zidovudine has not been shown to reduce the risk of HIV transmission to others.
3. Zidovudine is for oral administration only and must be taken every 4 hours around the clock.
4. Patients may continue to have illnesses associated with AIDS or ARC.

ADVERSE REACTIONS:
Most Frequent: Granulocytopenia and anemia. Also, headache, nausea, insomnia, myalgia.

DOSAGE:
Initially, 200 mg q 4 hr around the clock. If anemia or significant granulocytopenia occur, reduce dose or discontinue the drug.

Agents Used to Treat *Pneumocystis carinii* Pneumonitis

This section identifies the specific anti-infective agents used to treat *Pneumocystis carinii pneumonitis* (see also Appendix C).

PENTAMIDINE ISETHIONATE

MECHANISM OF ACTION:
Pentamidine is an antiprotozoal agent whose mode of action is not fully known; however, studies indicate that pentamidine inhibits the synthesis of DNA, RNA, phospholipids, and proteins.

INDICATIONS FOR USE:

Pentamidine is indicated for the treatment of *Pneumocystis carinii* pneumonia (PCP).

CONTRAINDICATIONS:

There are no contraindications for the use of this agent once the diagnosis of PCP has been established.

PRECAUTIONS:

1. Use with caution in patients with renal disease (accumulation may occur), hypertension, hypotension, hypoglycemia, hyperglycemia, leukopenia, thrombocytopenia, anemia, or hepatic impairment.
2. Monitor patient carefully for sudden, severe hypotension, hypoglycemia, cardiac arrhythmias, or other serious adverse effects.
3. Strict isolation techniques. (gown, cap, gloves, mask, goggles) should be used by health care providers to protect themselves when administering aerosolized medications to AIDS patients.

ADVERSE REACTIONS:

Most Serious: Leukopenia, hypoglycemia, thrombocytopenia, hypotension, acute renal failure, hypocalcemia, ventricular tachycardia, Stevens-Johnson syndrome. Death due to severe hypotension, hypoglycemia, cardiac arrhythmias.

Aerosol Administration: Bronchospasm, fatigue, severe cough (usually associated in patients with asthma or smoking), unpleasant taste, burning sensation in back of throat, mild hypoglycemia. Systemic side effects have not been noted with aerosol administration.

DOSAGE: ***IM, IV:*** 4 mg/kg/day in a single dose for 14 days. Dosage must be reduced in patients with renal failure.

Aerosol administration: Dissolve 600 mg of lypholized pentamidine with 6 ml of sterile water. Place solution in a specialized jet nebulizer (Respirgard II, Centimist, Aerotech II, etc.) and administer therapy for 20 to 30 minutes by nebulization. If bronchospasm occurs, reduce flow rate or administer a bronchodilator previous to pentamidine use.

TRIMETHOPRIM AND SULFAMETHOXAZOLE (TMP-SMZ)
BACTRIM, SEPTRA

MECHANISM OF ACTION:

The combination of trimethoprim and sulfamethoxazole effectively interferes with bacterial synthesis of essential nucleic acids and proteins.

INDICATIONS FOR USE:
Drug of choice in the treatment of pneumonia due to *P. carinii* in children and adults. Other uses include acute exacerbations of chronic bronchitis and acute otitis media caused by *H. influenzae* and *S. pneumoniae.* Also, shigellosis enteritis caused by *Shigella flexneri* and *Shigella sonnei.*

CONTRAINDICATIONS:
Hypersensitivity. Infants less than 2 months, pregnancy and lactation, megaloblastic anemia due to folate deficiency.

PRECAUTIONS:
1. This agent is not indicated to treat streptococcal pharyngitis.
2. Use with caution in the elderly and in patients with renal or hepatic impairment; increased adverse reactions may occur.
3. In patients with AIDS, an increased incidence of side effects is noted, such as rash, fever, and leukopenia.
4. Monitor patient for the occurrence of superinfection.

ADVERSE REACTIONS:
Most Common: Nausea, vomiting, anorexia, allergic skin rashes.
CNS: Headache, convulsions, hallucinations, vertigo, nervousness, apathy, mental depression.
GI: Nausea, vomiting, anorexia, stomatitis, abdominal pain, diarrhea, hepatitis, jaundice, pancreatitis.

DOSAGE: *IV:* 8 to 10 mg/kg given in divided doses every 6, 8, or 12 hours. For *P. carinii:* 15 to 20 mg/kg given in divided doses every 6 or 8 hours for up to 14 days.

Resuscitation Pharmacology and the American Heart Association's Advanced Cardiac Life Support Guidelines (ACLS) 19

This chapter focuses on the drugs commonly used during cardiopulmonary resuscitation (CPR). The goals of these pharmacologic agents are:

1. Correction of hypoxemia and acidosis.
2. Improvement of hemodynamics.
3. Suppression of ventricular tachycardia (V-tach) and/or ventricular fibrillation (V-fib).
4. Maintenance of coronary and cerebral perfusion to ultimately reestablish spontaneous circulation.
5. Optimization of cardiac function.

To enhance the learner's comprehension of the factors that interact with the primary resuscitation drugs, the basic arrhythmias with associated drug of choice used to correct the arrhythmia, a flow chart on understanding blood gas analysis, and ACLS algorithms are included at the end of this chapter (Figs. 19.1 to 19.9).

The first priority of CPR is early intervention; this consists of defibrillation in adults and ventilatory support in infants. Chest compression, assisted ventilation, and pharmacologic intervention are implemented to facilitate circulatory and ventilatory function, with the primary goal being to reestablish spontaneous cardiopulmonary dynamics. Once a stable rhythm and ventilatory pattern (with mechanical ventilation if necessary) have been established, pressors (such as catecholamines) are used to maintain circulation.

Of essential importance during cardiopulmonary resuscitation (along with endotracheal intubation) is the accessibility for drug administration. Intravenous drug administration is the preferred route, with the brachial vein being the site of choice for the placement of the IV line. If the intravenous route is not immediately accessible, endotracheal administration of certain drugs (e.g., epinephrine, atropine) may be utilized; however, the upper range of the IV dose must be given to elicit the same pharmacologic response as that of the IV route. Other drugs, such as lidocaine and bretylium, may also be administered endotracheally, yet hopefully an IV route has been established by the time these drugs are necessary, since they are not generally used during the first sequence of CPR.

PRIMARY RESUSCITATION DRUGS

OXYGEN

ACTIONS:
Supplemental oxygen is an essential drug during CPR. Oxygen delivery to organs and tissues is highly compromised during cardiopulmonary arrest. Severe hypoxemia in the compromised patient leads to anaerobic metabolism, lactic acid accumulation, and acidosis. Even with properly performed chest compressions, only 25 to 35% of the normal cardiac output is maintained. Therefore, oxygen delivery to the tissues is severely impaired. Irreversible cell death may occur if supplemental oxygen is not provided immediately. Oxygen administration elevates and maintains alveolar and arterial oxygen tension and content, thereby facilitating maximal tissue oxygenation.

INDICATIONS:
1. Cardiopulmonary arrest.
2. Shock states.
3. Cardiac or pulmonary impaired patients when hypoxemia or hypoxia is present.
4. Poisoning or toxic states in which respiratory depression, acidosis, or decreased levels of consciousness are present.
5. Sickle cell anemia crisis.

DOSAGE:
When available, 100% oxygen (via manual resuscitator) is given to all patients during cardiac arrest. Once an endotracheal tube has been established, oxygen may be more effectively delivered directly to the lungs. There are no contraindications to 100% oxygen delivery in the short time period required for resuscitation.

EPINEPHRINE

ACTIONS:
Epinephrine's potent pharmacologic action produces both α- and β-adrenergic responses. Epinephrine's sympathomimetic effects increase:

Heart rate
Myocardial contractile force
Myocardial oxygen consumption
Myocardial tone (e.g., converts fine V-fib to coarse V-fib).
Systemic vascular tone
Arterial blood pressure

The arterial and peripheral vasoconstricting effects of α stimulation increases aortic diastolic pressure, which facilitates coronary and cerebral perfusion pressure and ultimately coronary and cerebral blood flow.

The β-adrenergic effects, during CPR, are not necessarily indicated; however, epinephrine is still the drug of choice during CPR rather than pure α-adrenergic drugs because pure α-adrenergic drugs do not enhance and support cerebral blood flow to the same extent as epinephrine does.

INDICATIONS:
1. Drug of choice for anaphylactic shock and cardiac arrest.
2. For use during the resuscitation effort.
3. Antidote of choice for histamine overdose and allergic reactions.
4. Stokes-Adams syndrome.

DOSAGE:
For cardiac arrest: 0.5 to 1 mg (5 to 10 ml of 1:10,000 solution).
During resuscitation effort: 0.5 mg up to 1 mg (1:10,000 solution) given IV, repeated every 5 minutes as needed. May also be administered via endotracheal tube (1 to 2 mg in 10 ml distilled water) if IV route has not been established. Must stop chest compressions while instilling epinephrine into the endotracheal tube.
Pediatric: 0.01 mg/kg of 1:10,000 solution (0.1 ml/kg) given IV, ET, or IC.

ATROPINE

ACTIONS:
Atropine is a parasympatholytic drug that acts to accelerate the rate of sinus node discharge, improves atrioventricular (AV) conduction by inhibiting vagal tone, and may restore cardiac rhythm by initiating electrical activity during asystolic cardiac arrest (see also Chapter 9).

INDICATIONS:

1. Sinus bradycardia with accompanied hemodynamic compromised hypotension, ventricular ectopy, and/or myocardial ischemia.
2. Ventricular asystole.

DOSAGE:

For patients with asystole: 1 mg IV, repeated once if necessary.
Endotracheal administration: 1 to 2 mg diluted with 10 ml sterile water or normal saline.
For symptomatic bradycardia: Range; 0.4 to 1.0 mg, repeated every 1 to 2 hours as needed, up to a maximum dose of 2 mg. Lower doses (<0.4 mg) may cause rebound vagotonic effects (e.g., bradycardia), which may precipitate ventricular fibrillation.
Pediatric: 0.02 mg/kg IV or ET. Minimum dose 0.1 mg; maximum dose 1.0 mg. May be repeated in 5 minutes.

LIDOCAINE

ACTIONS:

Lidocaine is the antiarrhythmic drug of choice for ventricular ectopy. Lidocaine suppresses ventricular arrhythmias (V-tach, V-fib) by elevating the ventricular threshold, and also terminates reentrant arrhythmias by supressing myocardial conduction.

INDICATIONS:

1. Ventricular tachycardia, fibrillation.
2. Premature ventricular complexes (PVCs) in the critically ill patient and in patients in whom PVCs are associated with myocardial ischemia or infarction.
3. Prophylaxis against V-fib.

DOSAGE:

For V-tach or V-fib: 1 mg/kg IV bolus. Once given, defibrillation should be reattempted. Repetitive doses of 0.5 mg/kg, up to a total dose of 3 mg/kg may be given every 8 to 10 minutes, or a second bolus of 1 mg/kg may be given.
Pediatric: 1 mg/kg/dose IV bolus.
For primary prophylaxis against V-fib: Initial bolus of 1.5 mg/kg followed by continuous infusion at 2 to 4 mg/min. Reduce dose by 50% in patients with impaired hepatic blood flow (acute MI, CHF, or shock).

PROCAINAMIDE

ACTIONS:

Procainamide suppresses ventricular ectopy and effectively terminates reentrant dysrhythmias by slowing ventricular conduction and by prolonging the refractory period of ventricular tissue.

INDICATIONS:

1. For persistent V-fib.
2. Suppression of PVCs, recurrent V-tach not controlled by lidocaine.

DOSAGE:

100 mg every 5 minutes at a rate of 20 mg/min until one of the following occurs: hypotension, widening of the QRS complex by 50%, suppression of the arrhythmia, or administration of a total of 1 g.

BRETYLIUM TOSYLATE

ACTIONS:

Bretylium is an antiarrhythmic agent that has both adrenergic and direct myocardial effects. Bretylium causes the early release of norepinephrine from the adrenergic postganglionic nerve terminals. In addition, bretylium inhibits norepinephrine release from peripheral adrenergic sites. Initially, hypertension, tachycardia, and in some an increase in the cardiac output is noted; then orthostatic hypotension occurs from these effects. Bretylium also prevents the reuptake of norepinephrine, thereby potentiating the effects of exogenously administered catecholamines.

Bretylium produces a positive inotropic effect on the myocardium. It elevates the ventricular fibrillation threshold and also increases the action potential duration and effective refractory period in the heart, which may act to terminate reentrant dysrhythmias.

INDICATIONS:

V-tach or V-fib that is refractory to lidocaine, procainamide, or repeated shocks. Bretylium is not indicated as first-line treatment during cardiopulmonary resuscitation efforts.

DOSAGE:

For V-fib: 5 mg/kg undiluted bretylium, given by rapid IV infusion.

For persistent V-fib: Increase dose to 10 mg/kg, repeated at 15- to 30-minute intervals, up to a maximum dose of 30 mg/kg.

For refractory or recurrent V-tach: 500 mg (10 ml) diluted to 50 ml and 5 to 10 mg/kg injected IV, given over a period of 8 to 10 minutes.

SODIUM BICARBONATE

ACTIONS:

Sodium bicarbonate is used in the management of the *metabolic* component of acidosis. Metabolic acidosis results from anerobic metabolism and the production of lactic acid during inadequate tissue oxygenation. Sodium bicarbonate buffers metabolic acidosis by reacting with hydrogen ions to form water and carbon dioxide. However, the high carbon dioxide content of sodium bicarbonate may worsen intracellular hypercarbia and acidosis. Also, studies have shown that sodium bicarbonate administration during resuscitation efforts does not enhance ventricular defibrillation, improve spontaneous circulation, or facilitate survival in the cardiac arrest patient. Therefore, recent guidelines of the American Heart Association recommends that sodium bicarbonate not be administered during the resuscitation effort; or if it is administered, it should be done only after defibrillation, chest compression, endotracheal intubation, vigorous hyperventilation (to reduce and correct acidosis) with 100% oxygen, and the administration of drugs such as epinephrine and lidocaine, or if pre-existing metabolic acidosis has been documented.

INDICATIONS:

Lack of proof of efficacy of this drug has led to its not being recommended during cardiopulmonary resuscitation by the American Heart Association. Its use is indicated only if preexisting metabolic acidosis has been documented.

DOSAGE:

If given: 1 mEq/kg initially, then a maximum of ½ the initial dose administered not more often than every 10 minutes.

CALCIUM

ACTIONS:

Calcium produces a positive inotropic effect on the myocardium that tends to increase myocardial contractile force and ventricular automaticity.

INDICATIONS:

This drug is indicated during cardiopulmonary resuscitation for its inotropic effect only when the administration of epinephrine has failed to produce desired results, or in cardiac arrest patients who show acute hyperkalemia, hypocalcemia, or calcium channel blocker toxicity.

DOSAGE:
Calcium chloride (preferred): 2 to 4 mg/kg of 10% solution (500 mg to 1 g IV), may be repeated at 10-minute intervals.
Pediatric: 0.15 ml/kg.
Calcium gluceptate: 5 to 7 ml.
Calcium gluconate: 5 to 8 ml.
NOTE: Rapid IV injection may slow the heart rate.

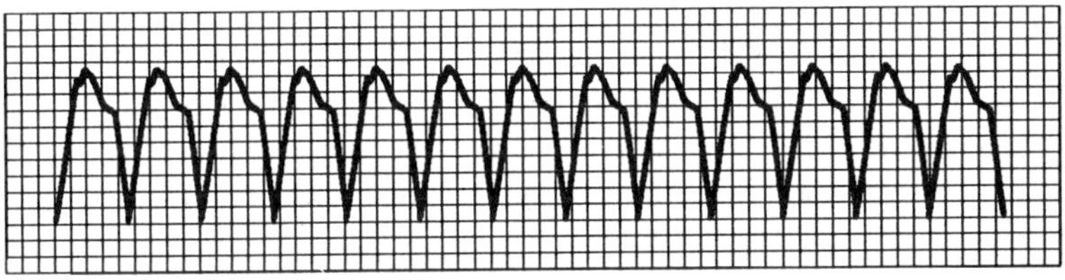

Figure 19.1. Ventricular tachycardia. Ventricular rate ranges from 50 (slow ventricular tachycardia) to 220 (rapid ventricular tachycardia) P waves, ST segments, and T waves are obscured by the QRS complexes, which are wide and bizarre. R-R interval is usually regular. Treatment includes lidocaine, and if the onset of V-tach is witnessed a precordial thump is given. Direct-current shock (up to 360 joules) is applied if the patient is rapidly deteriorating.

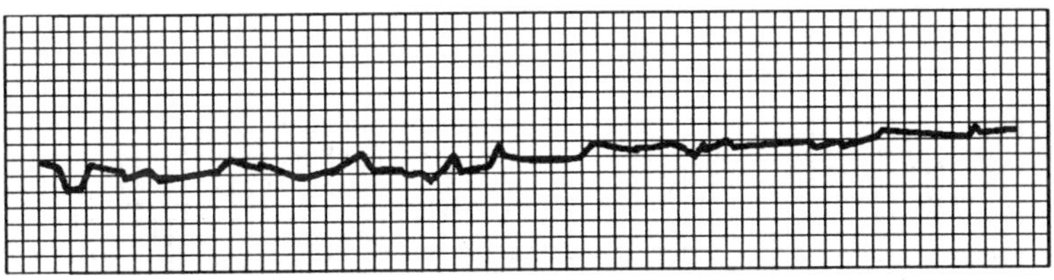

Figure 19.2. Ventricular fibrillation. Ventricular rate is rapid and chaotic, lacking a pattern. Cardiac output is inadequate. Treatment includes immediate direct-current shock (up to 360 joules), lidocaine, and the initiation of cardiopulmonary resuscitation if defibrillation is not effective.

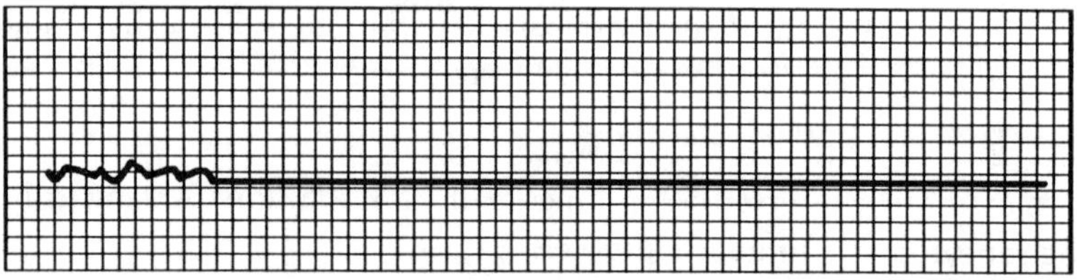

Figure 19.3. Cardiac arrest or asystole. It is caused by complete, acute heart failure. Treatment consists of cardiopulmonary resuscitation: intubation, ventilation, closed chest compressions, epinephrine.

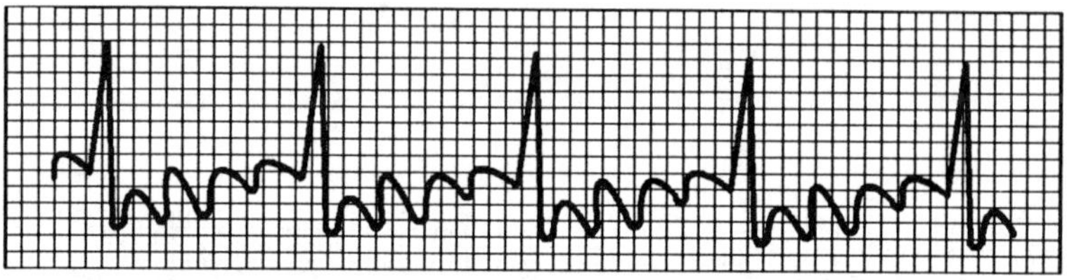

Figure 19.4. Atrial flutter. Atrial rate ranges from 250 and 350 beats per minute. QRS complexes are usually narrow. P waves are superimposed upon T waves (forming F waves) and resemble a "sawtooth" pattern. Treatment includes digitalis or quinidine, elective cardioversion (20 to 50 w/sec) or a temporary pacemaker.

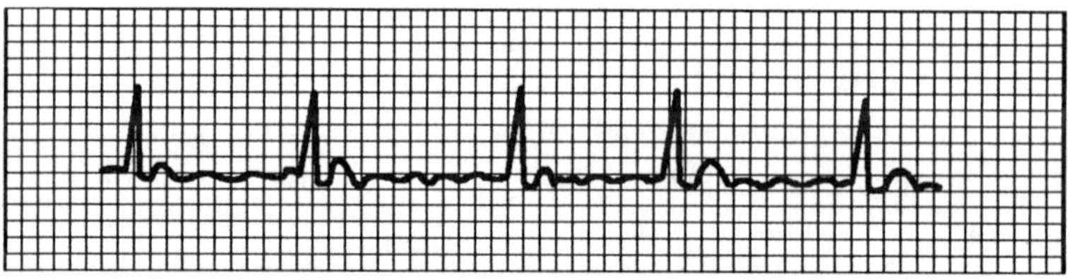

Figure 19.5. Atrial fibrillation. Atrial rate ranges from 350 to 500 beats per minute (but may reach as high as 700 beats per minute). The fibrillatory (or f) waves cause a varying, constantly changing atrial rate. ST segments and T waves will vary. Treatment includes digitalis or quinidine and elective cardioversion or a temporary pacemaker (for low ventricular rates due to block).

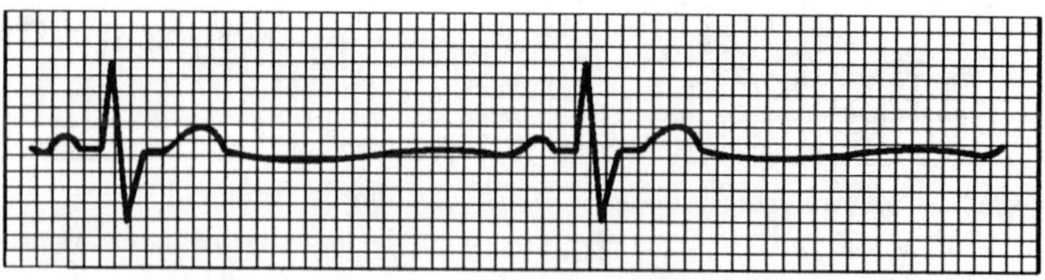

Figure 19.6. Sinus bradycardia. Rate <60 beats per minute. When accompanied with hypotension, poor cardiac output, or heart failure, may treat with atropine or temporary pacemaker (for low output rates).

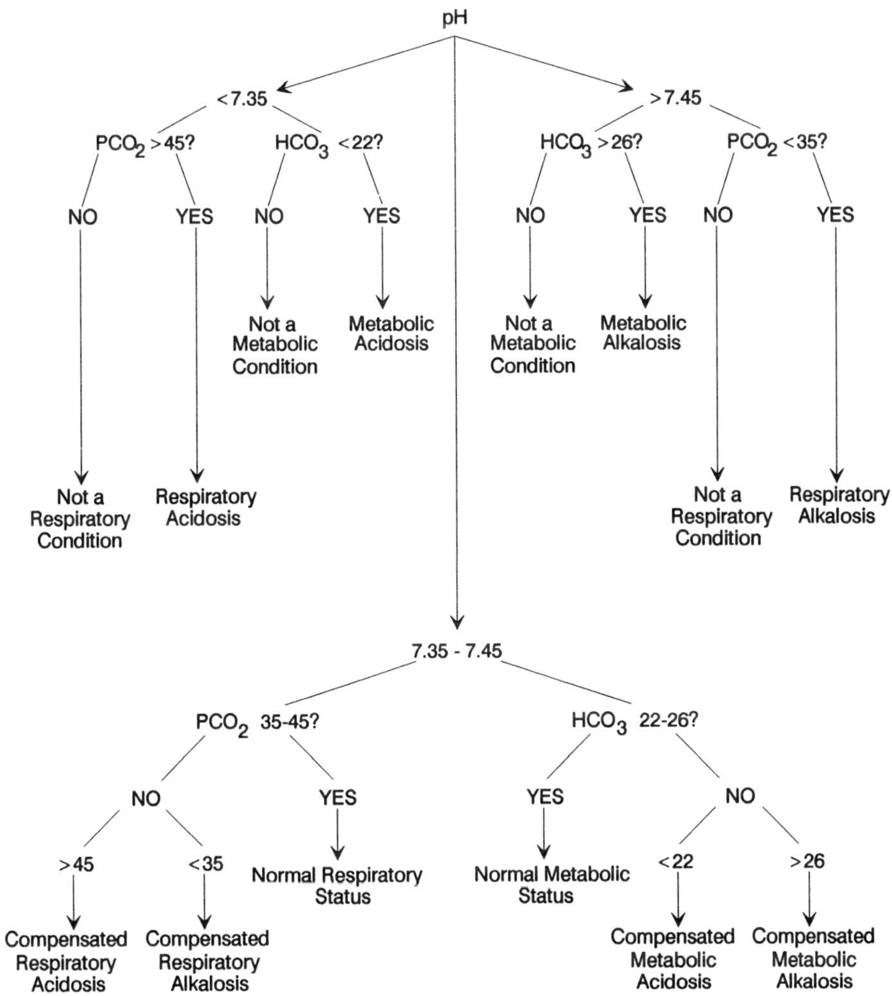

CLASSIFICATION OF HYPOXEMIA

Mild	Moderate	Severe
PaO_2 60-79 mmHg	PaO_2 40-59 mmHg	PaO_2 <40 mmHg

Figure 19.7. Understanding arterial blood gases.

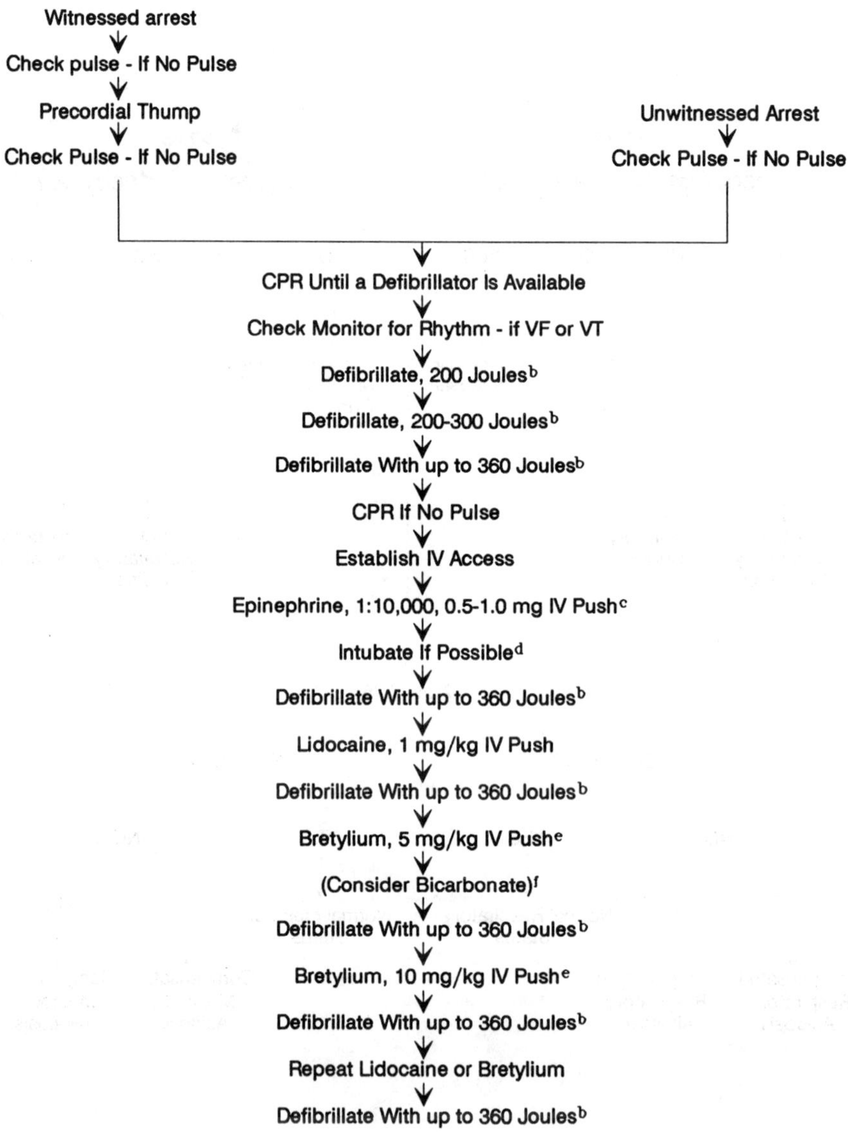
Witnessed arrest
Check pulse - If No Pulse
Precordial Thump
Check Pulse - If No Pulse
Unwitnessed Arrest
Check Pulse - If No Pulse
CPR Until a Defibrillator Is Available
Check Monitor for Rhythm - if VF or VT
Defibrillate, 200 Joules[b]
Defibrillate, 200-300 Joules[b]
Defibrillate With up to 360 Joules[b]
CPR If No Pulse
Establish IV Access
Epinephrine, 1:10,000, 0.5-1.0 mg IV Push[c]
Intubate If Possible[d]
Defibrillate With up to 360 Joules[b]
Lidocaine, 1 mg/kg IV Push
Defibrillate With up to 360 Joules[b]
Bretylium, 5 mg/kg IV Push[e]
(Consider Bicarbonate)[f]
Defibrillate With up to 360 Joules[b]
Bretylium, 10 mg/kg IV Push[e]
Defibrillate With up to 360 Joules[b]
Repeat Lidocaine or Bretylium
Defibrillate With up to 360 Joules[b]

Figure 19.8. Ventricular fibrillation (and pulseless ventricular tachycardia).[A] This sequence was developed to assist in teaching how to treat a broad range of patients with ventricular fibrillation (VF) or pulseless ventricular tachycardia (VT). Some patients may require care not specified herein. This algorithm should not be construed as prohibiting such flexibility. Flow of algorithm presumes that VF is continuing. CPR indicates cardiopulmonary resuscitation. Reproduced with permission. *Textbook of Advanced Cardiac Life Support,* 1987. Copyright American Heart Association.

[a]Pulseless VT should be treated identically to VF.

[b]Check pulse and rhythm after each shock. If VF recurs after transiently converting (rather than persists without ever converting), use whatever energy level has previously been successful for defibrillation.

[c]Epinephrine should be repeated every five minutes.

[d]Intubation is preferable. If it can be accompanied simultaneously with other techniques, then the earlier the better. However, defibrillation and epinephrine are more important initially if the patient can be ventilated without intubation.

[e]Some may prefer repeated doses of lidocaine, which may be given in 0.5 mg/kg boluses every eight minutes to a total dose of 3 mg/kg.

[f]Value of sodium bicarbonate is questionable during cardiac arrest, and it is not recommended for routine cardiac arrest sequence. Consideration of its use in a dose of 1 mEq/kg is appropriate at this point. Half of original dose may be repeated every ten minutes if it is used.

If Rhythm Is Unclear and Possibly Ventricular Fibrillation, Defibrillate as for VF. If Asystole is Present[a]

↓

Continue CPR

↓

Establish IV Access

↓

Epinephrine, 1:10,000, 0.5-1.0 mg IV Push[b]

↓

Intubate When Possible[c]

↓

Atropine, 1.0 mg IV Push (Repeated in 5 min)

↓

(Consider Bicarbonate)[d]

↓

Consider Pacing

Figure 19.9. Asystole (cardiac standstill). This sequence was developed to assist in teaching how to treat a broad range of patients with asystole. Some patients may require care not specified herein. This algorithm should not be construed to prohibit such flexibility. Flow of algorithm presumes asystole is continuing. VF indicates ventricular fibrillation; IV, intravenous. Reproduced with permission. *Textbook of Advanced Cardiac Life Support,* 1987. Copyright American Heart Association.

[a]Asystole should be confirmed in two leads.

[b]Epinephrine should be repeated every five minutes.

[c]Intubation is preferable; if it can be accomplished simultaneously with other techniques, then the earlier the better. However, cardiopulmonary resuscitation (CPR) and use of epinephrine are more important initially if patient can be ventilated without intubation. (Endotracheal epinephrine may be used.)

[d]Value of sodium bicarbonate is questionable during cardiac arrest, and it is not recommended for the routine cardiac arrest sequence. Consideration of its use in a dose of 1 mEq/kg is appropriate at this point. Half of original dose may be repeated every ten minutes if it is used.

CRITICAL CARE DRUGS 20

The primary purpose of this chapter is to familiarize the practitioner with some of the more commonly used diuretics and cardiovascular drugs.

Note: Drugs that have already been presented in previous chapters (e.g., atropine, lidocaine, epinephrine, morphine, Narcan, Pavulon, etc.) are not presented again. Please see the index for a page number when referring to these drugs.

DIURETIC AGENTS

Diuretic agents have the ability to facilitate urinary output of water and sodium by enhancing the normal function of the kidney. This is done by one of three primary mechanisms:

1. Increase the glomerular filtration rate.
2. Decrease sodium reabsorption by the renal tubules.
3. Induce and promote the excretion of sodium by the kidney.

Classification of a diuretic agent is based on its primary mechanism of action. An example from each category is given, followed by a listing of related diuretics.

Carbonic Anhydrase Inhibitors

ACETAZOLAMIDE
DIAMOX

ACTIONS:

Carbonic anhydrase is an enzyme that catalyzes the union of CO_2 and water to form carbonic acid (H_2CO_3), which dissociates into free hydrogen and bicarbonate. Acetazolamide inhibits the action of carbonic anhydrase, thereby preventing hydrogen ion formation and secretion in the renal tubule, which then causes increased excretion of sodium, potassium, bicarbonate, and water. The total diuretic action of acetazolamide is hindered by the development of tolerance due to its promotion of metabolic acidosis through depletion of bicarbonate.

INDICATIONS:

1. Edema due to CHF.
2. Drug-induced edema.
3. Treatment of hyperkalemic periodic paralysis.
4. Acute mountain sickness after exposure to high altitude.

CONTRAINDICATIONS:

Hypersensitivity to this drug. Decreased sodium or potassium levels, moderate renal and hepatic disease, hyperchloremic acidosis, electrolyte imbalance, severe COPD patients, severe or absolute glaucoma.

PRECAUTIONS:

1. Increasing the dosage does not increase diuresis. It may actually act to decrease diuresis.
2. Electrolyte imbalance should be corrected before administration of this drug.
3. Acetazolamide may aggravate acidosis, therefore use with extreme caution in patients with severe degrees of respiratory acidosis.

ADVERSE REACTIONS:

CNS: Convulsions, fatigue, nervousness, sedation, depression, confusion, headache, vertigo, paresthesias of the extremities.

GI: Vomiting, nausea, constipation, anorexia.

Miscellaneous: Weight loss, fever, acidosis (may be corrected by administering bicarbonate).

DOSAGE:

For edema due to CHF or drug-related edema: 250 to 375 mg (5 mg/kg) once daily for 1 or 2 days.

Other Carbonic Anhydrase Inhibitors

Dichlorphenamide (Daranide).

Thiazide Diuretics

CHLOROTHIAZIDE
DIURIL, DIACHLOR, DIURIGEN

ACTIONS:
Chlorothiazide is a thiazide diuretic that increases the excretion of sodium and chloride (with a corresponding loss of water) by decreasing the rate of sodium and chloride reabsorption by the distal renal tubules. Other effects include increased potassium excretion, uric acid retention, and reduced calcium excretion. Onset of action occurs within 1 to 2 hours with a duration of 6 to 12 hours.

INDICATIONS:
1. Used in conjunction with other diuretics in patients with edema associated with CHF, patients with hepatic cirrhosis, and patients with edema due to renal impairment (nephrotic syndrome, acute glomerulonephritis, and chronic renal failure).
2. Hypertension; this drug may be used alone or with other hypotensive agents to enhance their effectiveness.

CONTRAINDICATIONS:
Hypersensitivity to thiazides, anuria, renal decompensation.

PRECAUTIONS:
1. IV administration is indicated only when oral medication cannot be taken or in acute emergencies.
2. Monitor fluid and electrolyte balance for the precipitation of hepatic coma in patients with hepatic impairment or progressive liver disease.
3. This agent may increase the toxic effects of lithium.
4. Episodes of apnea may occur with concurrent use with nondepolarizing muscle relaxants (possibly due to potentiating effects and hypokalemia).

ADVERSE REACTIONS:
CNS: Dizziness, vertigo, headache, paresthesias, syncope, anxiety, depression.
Cardiovascular: Orthostatic hypotension, PVCs, palpitations.
Pulmonary: Sore throat, congestion, cough, respiratory distress, possibly with pneumonitis.
GI: Nausea, vomiting, abdominal pain, diarrhea, pancreatitis, cholecystitis, jaundice.

OVERDOSAGE:
Symptoms include electrolyte imbalance, potassium depletion, nausea, vomiting, hypotension, apnea, coma. Treatment consists of gastric lavage (prevent aspiration), monitoring of electrolyte balance, and cardiopulmonary support if necessary.

DOSAGE:
For edema: 0.5 to 2 g once or twice daily orally or IV. IV route not recommended unless oral medication is not feasible or for emergency situations.
For hypertension: 0.5 to 2 g daily (oral route only).

Other Thiazides and Related Diuretics

Hydrochlorothiazide (Esidrix, Oretic, Diaqua, Hydro-T), bendroflumethiazide (Naturetin), cyclothiazide (Anhydron), methyclothiazide (Enduron, Ethon, Aquatensen), benzthiazide (Aquatag, Exna, Hydrex, Marazide, Proaqua), hydroflumethiazide (Diucardin, Saluron), trichlormethiazide (Metahydrin, Naqua, Diurese, Trichlorex), polythiazide (Renese), quinethazone (Hydromox), metolazone (Diulo, Zaroxolyn, Mycrox), chlorthalidone (Hygroton, Hylidone, Thalitone), indapamide (Lozol).

Loop Diuretics

FUROSEMIDE
LASIX

ACTIONS:
Furosemide is a potent diuretic agent that inhibits the reabsorption of sodium and chloride in the ascending loop of Henle and in the proximal and distal tubules. In addition, furosemide promotes the excretion of potassium, magnesium, calcium, and, to a lesser extent, bicarbonate. The onset of action of orally administered furosemide is within 60 minutes with a duration of 6 to 8 hours. The onset of action of intravenously administered furosemide is within 5 minutes with a duration of 2 hours.

INDICATIONS:
1. Edema associated with CHF, hepatic cirrhosis, renal disease.
2. Used as an adjuvant in acute pulmonary edema.
3. Hypertension (orally administered).

CONTRAINDICATIONS:
Hypersensitivity to furosemide, anuria.

PRECAUTIONS:
1. IV administration is indicated when a rapid onset of action is preferred (e.g., acute pulmonary edema), when GI absorption is impaired, or when oral administration is not feasible.
2. Monitor patient for signs of dehydration. Rapid and excessive weight loss may potentiate an acute hypotensive crisis.
3. If given in excessive amounts, furosemide may cause electrolyte depletion. Monitor patient for hyponatremia, hypochloremic alkalosis, hypokalemia.
4. Coadministration of aminoglycosides may increase the potential for ototoxicity.

ADVERSE REACTIONS:
CNS: Paresthesia, restlessness, xanthopsia, headache, vertigo, dizziness.
Cardiovascular: Orthostatic hypotension.
GI: Anorexia, nausea, vomiting, cramping, diarrhea, constipation, pancreatitis, jaundice.

OVERDOSAGE:
Profound water loss and electrolyte depletion, dehydration, circulatory collapse. Treatment consists of supportive measures and replacement of fluid and electrolyte loss.

DOSAGE:
Edema: Oral dose ranges from 20 to 80 mg/day up to 600 mg/day in patients with severe edema. IM, IV: 20 to 40 mg up to 80 mg for acute pulmonary edema.
Hypertension: Oral administration only, 40 mg twice daily.

Other Loop Diuretics

Ethacrynic acid (Edecrin), bumetanide (Bumex).

Osmotic Diuretics

MANNITOL
OSMITROL

ACTIONS:
Mannitol is an osmotic diuretic that inhibits the reabsorption of sodium and water in the proximal tubules, the loop of Henle, and the collecting duct. This

effect is brought about by mannitol's ability to elevate the osmotic pressure of the glomerular filtrate, thereby impeding the reabsorption of water in the renal tubules. By this action, the excretion not only of water, but also of sodium and chloride, is increased. The onset of intravenously administered mannitol is within 60 minutes with a duration of 6 to 8 hours.

INDICATIONS:

1. In the treatment or prevention of acute renal failure.
2. Reduction of intracranial pressure and cerebral edema.
3. Reduction of intraocular pressure.
4. As a diagnostic tool to measure the glomerular filtration rate.

CONTRAINDICATIONS:

Severe pulmonary congestion, severe dehydration, anuria due to severe renal disease.

PRECAUTIONS:

1. Serious electrolyte imbalance may occur with excessive use.
2. Patient's cardiovascular system must be carefully monitored before rapid administration of mannitol due to the prompt expansion of extracellular fluid and the potential of developing fulminating congestive heart failure and pulmonary edema.

ADVERSE REACTIONS:

CNS: Headache, convulsions, dizziness.

Cardiovascular: Hypotension, hypertension, edema, tachycardia, chest pain.

Pulmonary: Pulmonary congestion, edema.

GI: Nausea, vomiting, diarrhea.

OVERDOSAGE:

Symptoms consist of orthostatic tachycardia, hypotension, polyuria, stupor, convulsions, hyponatremia. Treatment includes supportive care to correct fluid and electrolyte imbalance, discontinuing the drug, and hemodialysis if necessary to clear mannitol.

DOSAGE:

IV: Usual adult dose, 50 to 200 g/day (administration rate is adjusted to maintain a urine flow of at least 30 to 50 ml/hr).

To reduce intracranial pressure: 1.5 to 2 g/kg of a 15%, 20%, or 25% solution given slowly over 30 to 60 minutes.

Prevention of acute renal failure: 50 to 100 g as a 5% to 25% solution given during cardiovascular or other types of surgery.

Other Osmotic Diuretics

Urea (Ureaphil), glycerin (Glyrol, Osmoglyn).

Potassium-Sparing Diuretics

SPIRONOLACTONE
ALATONE, ALDACTONE

ACTIONS:

Spironolactone blocks sodium reabsorption in the distal tubule by competitively inhibiting the actions of the aldosterone receptors. Potassium is normally exchanged for sodium in the distal tubule and then secreted into the urine. By preventing the potassium-sodium exchange, potassium is spared from secretion.

INDICATIONS:

1. Essential hypertension (in combination with other drugs).
2. Hypokalemia.
3. Management of edema and sodium retention in the CHF patient.
4. Cirrhosis of the liver when accompanied by edema or ascites.

CONTRAINDICATIONS:

Anuria, acute renal failure, hyperkalemia.

PRECAUTIONS:

1. Patient must be carefully monitored for possible fluid and electrolyte imbalances.
2. Spironolactone may induce or aggravate hyponatremia.
3. Coadministered potassium preparations may result in hyperkalemia, resulting in an increased risk of cardiac arrhythmias or cardiac arrest.
4. The absorption rate of spironolactone is increased when administered with food.
5. May produce drowsiness; observe caution when driving or operating machinery that requires alertness.
6. Potassium-sparing diuretics are generally used in combination with thiazides and loop diuretics to enhance these drugs' actions and effects and to overcome the kaliuretic effect produced by these agents.

ADVERSE REACTIONS:

GI: Cramping, diarrhea, gastric bleeding, vomiting.

CNS: Drowsiness, lethargy, headache, mental confusion, ataxia.

Miscellaneous: Thirst, skin rash, hyperchloremic metabolic acidosis in decompensated hepatic cirrhosis.

DOSAGE:

Edema: range, 25 to 200 mg/day. *Essential hypertension:* Initially, 50 to 100 mg/day. *Hypokalemia:* 25 to 100 mg/day.

Other Potassium-Sparing Diuretics

Amiloride (Midamor), triamterene (Dyrenium). These agents are not aldosterone inhibitors as is spironolactone, but act directly on the distal tubule to inhibit sodium reabsorption.

THE ANTICONVULSANT AGENTS

PHENYTOIN SODIUM
DILANTIN

ACTIONS:

Phenytoin is an anticonvulsant agent that inhibits seizure activity at the motor cortex level. Phenytoin promotes the efflux of sodium from neurons, thereby stabilizing the threshold against hyperexcitability. Phenytoin is preferred over phenobarbital in the adult; however, because of phenytoin's adverse reactions, phenobarbital is the drug of first choice in children and infants. Phenytoin and phenobarbital are occasionally used together when a single drug is ineffective in controlling seizures.

INDICATIONS:

1. Control of grand mal and psychomotor seizures.
2. Prevention and treatment of seizures occurring during or after neurosurgery.
3. Control of status epilepticus of the grand mal type.
4. Unlabeled use: antiarrhythmic agent useful in digitalis-induced arrhythmias.

CONTRAINDICATIONS:

Hypersensitivity, sinus bradycardia, sinoatrial block, second- or third-degree AV block (phenytoin depresses spontaneous depolarization in ventricular tissues).

PRECAUTIONS:

1. Abrupt withdrawal of this drug may induce status epilepticus.
2. Not indicated for seizures due to hypoglycemia.

3. Use with caution in patients with impaired hepatic function.

ADVERSE REACTIONS:

CNS: Ataxia, confusion, dizziness, insomnia, nervousness, diplopia, irritability, depression, tremor, headache.

Cardiovascular: Cardiovascular collapse, CNS depression, hypotension (occurs when drug is rapidly infused).

GI: Nausea, vomiting, diarrhea, constipation.

Miscellaneous: Toxic hepatitis, liver damage, hyperglycemia, chest pain, edema, fever, pulmonary fibrosis, acute pneumonitis.

OVERDOSAGE:

Mean lethal dose is 2 to 5 g. Death is due to respiratory and circulatory depression. No known antidote is available. Hemodialysis may be necessary in severe intoxication.

DOSAGE:

PO: 300 mg daily in divided doses. Maintenance dose includes 300 to 400 mg/day up to a maximum of 600 mg/day.

IV: Loading dose of 15 mg/kg, then 5 mg/kg given after 12 hours from loading dose. Not to exceed an infusion rate of 50 mg/min.

PHENOBARBITAL

ACTIONS:

Phenobarbital is a long-acting barbiturate that is effective not only as a sedative, but also as an anticonvulsant. Phenobarbital decreases motor activity by depressing impulses to the sensory cortex.

INDICATIONS:

1. Generalized tonic-clonic (grand mal) seizures and partial (focal motor or sensory) seizures.
2. For emergent control of acute convulsive episodes such as status epilepticus, eclampsia, cerebral hemorrhage, meningitis, tetanus, and toxic reactions to strychnine or local anesthetics.

Note: For contraindications, precautions, and adverse reactions, refer to Chapter 16.

DOSAGE:

PO: 50 to 100 mg 2 to 3 times daily. Children: 15 to 50 mg 2 to 3 times daily.

IM, IV: 200 to 300 mg, repeated after 6 hr if necessary. Maximum 1 to 2 g in a 24-hour period. Children (IV only): 20 mg/kg, then 6 mg/kg q 20 min, prn. Maximum 40 mg/kg/24 hours.

Other Anticonvulsant Agents

Mephenytoin (Mesantoin), ethotoin (Peganone), ethosuximide (Zarontin), methsuximide (Celontin Kapseals), phensuximide (Milontin Kapseals), paramethadione (Paradione), trimethadione (Tridione), primidone (Mysoline, Myidone), valproic acid (Deproic, Depakene, Depakote), carbamazepine (Tegretol, Epitol), phenacemide (Phenurone). Paraldehyde, magnesium sulfate, acetazolamide, and selected benzodiazepines (Clonazepam, Clorazepate, diazepam) are also used as anticonvulsant agents.

ANTIARRHYTHMIC AGENTS

DIGITALIS

ACTIONS:

Digitalis is an antiarrhythmic agent that produces both direct and indirect inotropic effects on the myocardium. Direct effects include increased myocardial contractility, increased refractory time period of the AV node, and increased peripheral resistance. Indirect actions include depression of the sinoatrial (SA) node and prolonged conduction to the AV node.

INDICATIONS:

1. Arrhythmias associated with congestive heart failure (CHF).
2. Atrial fibrillation; agent of choice to reduce ventricular rates and abolish the pulse deficit.
3. Atrial flutter.
4. Paroxysmal atrial tachycardia (PAT).

CONTRAINDICATIONS:

V-fib, V-tach, digitalis toxicity states, beriberi heart disease.

PRECAUTIONS:

1. Dosage must be adjusted in patients with renal insufficiency.
2. Existing conditions that may precipitate digitalis toxicity include hypokalemia, hypercalcemia, hypothyroidism, hypomagnesemia, alkalosis, and hypoxia. These conditions should be corrected before giving digitalis.
3. Do not administer IV calcium to patients receiving digitalis, since the effects of calcium on the myocardium are similar to those of digitalis.
4. All dosages are highly individualized.

ADVERSE REACTIONS—DIGITALIS TOXICITY

CNS: Headache, weakness, apathy, blurred vision, confusion, disorientation, seizures.

GI: Anorexia, nausea, vomiting, abdominal pain.

Cardiac Reactions: Multifocal ventricular premature complexes, nonparoxysmal AV junctional tachycardia, sinus irregularities and other dysrhythmias.

OVERDOSAGE:

Treatment of toxicity consists of discontinuing the drug, assessing serum potassium levels, and, if necessary, administering potassium chloride and/or an antiarrhythmic drug.

DOSAGE:

Loading dose: Total average dose 1.2 g (given in several equal doses q 6 hr).

Maintenance dose: 100 to 200 mg/day (range varies from 30 to 400 mg/day).

Other Cardiac (Digitalis) Glycosides

Glycoside mixtures, digitoxin (Crystodigin), deslanoside (Cedilanid-D), and digoxin (Lanoxin). Amrinone lactate (Inocor) is a positive inotropic agent that differs from the digitalis glycosides in that it inhibits phosphodiesterase activity on the myocardial cAMP system, thereby increasing cellular levels of cAMP. Amrinone's vasodilator activity is indicated for the short-term management of CHF and in patients not responsive to digitalis therapy or other conventional therapy (diuretics, vasodilators). Patients must be closely monitored for adverse reactions.

QUINIDINE SULFATE
CIN-QUIN, QUINIDEX

QUINIDINE GLUCONATE
DURAQUIN, QUINAGLUTE

QUINIDINE POLYGALACTURONATE
CARDIOQUIN

ACTIONS:

Quinidine's antiarrhythmic action depresses myocardial contractility, conduction velocity, excitability, and automaticity. It also increases the heart's refractory time period, thereby increasing the time interval in which the heart may respond to contraction. Quinidine's indirect anticholinergic effect acts to decrease vagal tone and enhance AV conduction.

INDICATIONS:

1. Oral: Premature atrial contractions, ventricular contractions, paroxysmal atrial tachycardia, paroxysmal and chronic A-fib, paroxysmal ventricular tachycardia (those not associated with complete heart block), paroxysmal AV junctional rhythm, A-flutter. Maintenance therapy after electrical conversion of A-fib or A-flutter.
2. Parenteral: Indicated when rapid effect is required or when oral therapy is not feasible.

CONTRAINDICATIONS:

Hypersensitivity to quinidine. Use with extreme caution in patients with subacute endocarditis, bradycardia, coronary occlusion, or extensive myocardial damage.

PRECAUTIONS:

1. Use with caution in patients with myasthenia gravis, acute infections, respiratory distress, asthma.
2. Monitor plasma quinidine levels frequently when doses of greater than 2 g/day are used.
3. Quinidine may not be effective if cholinergic drugs are used concurrently.
4. Quinidine's effects are diminished in the presence of hypokalemia and enhanced by potassium.
5. Elderly patients and patients with CHF or renal or hepatic impairments may require a reduced dosage.

ADVERSE REACTIONS:

CNS: Confusion, nervousness, headache, flushing, edema.

Cardiovascular: Bradycardia, heart block (partial or total), syncope, circulatory collapse, shock, widening of the QRS complex, cardiac asystole, ventricular ectopy.

GI: Nausea, vomiting, abdominal pain, diarrhea.

OVERDOSAGE:

Symptoms include lethargy, coma, respiratory arrest, seizures, tachyarrhythmias. Treatment consists of symptomatic support, respiratory intervention with assisted ventilations if necessary, ECG and blood pressure monitoring, and cardiac pacing if indicated.

DOSAGE:

Oral:

For premature atrial and ventricular contractions: 200 to 300 mg given up to 4 times daily.

For paroxysmal supraventricular contractions: 400 to 600 mg given q 2 to 3 hr until arrhythmia is suppressed.

Maintenance therapy: 200 to 300 mg given up to 4 times daily.

Sustained release forms: 300 to 600 mg q 8 to 12 hr.

Parenteral:

For parenteral use, patient must be continuously monitored for ECG changes. Parenteral use has, for the most part, been replaced by lidocaine or procainamide. IV: 330 mg or less of quinidine gluconate. May require up to 750 mg. IM: 600 mg quinidine gluconate initial dose for episodes of acute tachycardia. Then 400 mg as often as q 2 hr may be given.

VERAPAMIL HYDROCHLORIDE
CALAN, ISOPTIN

ACTIONS:

Verapamil is an antiarrhythmic, antianginal, antihypertensive calcium channel blocking agent (also referred to as a slow channel blocker or calcium antagonist) that has the ability to inhibit calcium ion transport across the myocardial cell membrane. This effect delays impulse transmission through the AV node, depresses myocardial contraction, and reduces spontaneous rhythm of sinus node. Increased coronary blood flow is noted along with increased oxygen supply to the myocardium. Verapamil also reduces myocardial oxygen demand by decreasing the heart rate and reducing afterload.

INDICATIONS:

1. For rapid conversion to sinus rhythm of paroxysmal supraventricular tachycardias. Onset of action is 2 to 3 minutes.
2. Temporary control to slow rapid ventricular rate in A-flutter or A-fib.
3. Angina pectoris due to coronary artery spasm.
4. Essential hypertension (oral route).

CONTRAINDICATIONS:

Hypersensitivity to verapamil. Cardiogenic shock, severe hypotension. Also, sick sinus syndrome (except with a functioning ventricular pacemaker), second- or third-degree AV block.

PRECAUTIONS:
1. Abrupt withdrawal of verapamil may cause chest pain.
2. Use with caution in patients with impaired renal and hepatic function.
3. Verapamil may increase the effects of nondepolarizing muscle relaxants and those of theophylline.
4. IV verapamil should not be used concomitantly (within a few hours) with β-adrenergic blocking agents. Both of these agents depress myocardial contractility and AV conduction.

ADVERSE REACTIONS:
CNS: Dizziness, nervousness, headache, fatigue, sleep disturbances.
Cardiovascular: Peripheral and pulmonary edema, tachycardia, palpitations, hypotension, syncope, third-degree AV block, bradycardia, CHF, MI.
GI: Nausea, vomiting, diarrhea, constipation, abdominal cramps.

OVERDOSAGE:
Symptoms include hypotension, bradycardia, decreased cardiac output, junctional rhythms, second- or third-degree AV block. Treatment consists of supportive care with IV fluids and Trendelenburg position (with hypotensive effects) and monitoring of cardiac and respiratory functions. β-Adrenergic agonists and IV calcium may be administered to counteract verapamil's effects.

DOSAGE:
PO: 240 to 480 mg/day. *IV:* 5 to 10 mg given by slow infusion over 2 minutes. 10 mg may be given additionally, if necessary, in 30 minutes. Maintenance dose of 0.005 mg/kg/min.

Other Antiarrhythmic Agents

Procainamide, lidocaine, bretylium (see Chapter 19), disopyramide (Napamide, Norpace), phenytoin (previously discussed), propranolol (refer to β-adrenergic blocking agents in this chapter), tocainide (Tonocard), mexiletine (Mexitil), flecainide (Tambocor), amiodarone (Cordarone).

ANTIANGINAL AGENTS

NIFEDIPINE
PROCARDIA

ACTIONS:
Nifedipine produces both coronary and peripheral arterial vasodilation. Nifedipine's actions are similar to those of verapamil in that it inhibits the

movement of calcium ions across the cellular membrane, thereby depressing both cardiac automaticity and conduction velocity.

INDICATIONS:

1. Hypertension.
2. Vasospastic (Prinzmetal's) angina.
3. Chronic stable angina refractory to nitrate therapy.
4. Nefedipine does not adversely affect respiratory function and may be used safely in asthmatics.

CONTRAINDICATIONS:

Hypersensitivity to nifedipine.

ADVERSE REACTIONS:

Refer to verapamil.

DOSAGE:

PO: Effective dosage range is 10 to 20 mg tid.

DILTIAZEM
CARDIZEM

ACTIONS:

Diltiazem's mode of action and effect are similar to those of verapamil. It has the ability to dilate coronary and peripheral arteries and arterioles and to depress SA and AV nodal functions by inhibiting the movement of calcium ions across the cell membrane.

INDICATIONS:

1. Angina pectoris due to coronary artery spasm.
2. Chronic stable angina.

CONTRAINDICATIONS:

Second- or third-degree heart block, hypotension (<90 mm Hg systolic), sick sinus syndrome (except with a functioning ventricular pacemaker).

ADVERSE REACTIONS:

Refer to verapamil.

DOSAGE:

Initially 30 mg qid, then may increase dosage gradually to 180 to 360 mg tid or qid at 1- to 2-day intervals until desired results are achieved.

NITROGLYCERIN
TRIDEL, NITROSTAT, NITRO-BID

ACTIONS:

Nitroglycerin is an antianginal, antihypertensive agent whose primary pharmacologic action is the relaxation and dilation of vascular smooth muscle of both arterial and venous vessels. Nitroglycerin improves coronary circulating blood flow, reduces myocardial oxygen consumption, and reduces systemic and peripheral vascular resistance and arterial pressure. Nitroglycerin's effect also reduces elevated central venous pressure, pulmonary capillary wedge pressure, and pulmonary vascular resistance.

INDICATIONS:

1. IV: For the control and prevention of hypertensive episodes due to surgical procedures, cardiovascular procedures, and coronary artery bypass surgery. Also, CHF associated with acute MI.
2. Sublingual: For the relief of acute anginal periods. To reduce the work of the heart in patients with acute MI or CHF.

CONTRAINDICATIONS:

Hypersensitivity to nitrates. Hypotension, uncorrected hypovolemia, acute or recent myocardial infarction, severe anemia, increased intracranial pressure.

PRECAUTIONS:

1. Excessive doses may produce severe headaches.
2. Additive hypotensive effects may be noted with concurrent use of other antihypertensive agents and β-adrenergic blockers.
3. Severe hypotension and cardiovascular collapse may result with concurrent use of alcohol.
4. Monitoring of the pulmonary capillary wedge pressure (PCWP) facilitates titration of the drug. A reduction in the PCWP usually precedes the onset of hypotension.
5. Use with caution in patients with severe hepatic or renal disease.

ADVERSE REACTIONS:

CNS: Headache (may be persistent and severe), dizziness, vertigo, restlessness, weakness.

Cardiovascular: Tachycardia, palpitations, syncope, collapse, hypotension, paradoxical bradycardia.

GI: Nausea, vomiting, abdominal pain.

Methemoglobinemia: High doses of nitrates may interfere with the normal conversion of methemoglobin back to hemoglobin.

OVERDOSAGE:

Symptoms include marked responses listed under adverse reactions. Treatment consists of IV fluids and monitoring of arterial blood gases and methemoglobin. Epinephrine administration is contraindicated in overdosage. The hemodynamic effects of nitroglycerin are of short duration and no further intervention should be necessary.

DOSAGE:

IV: Dose may be titrated until a response is observed. Start with 5 μg/min and titrate upward in 5 μg/min increments with increases every 3 to 5 minutes until a response is noted.

Sublingual: Dissolve 1 tablet under the tongue at the first sign of an acute anginal attack. Do not exceed 3 tablets in 15 minutes.

Other Antianginal Agents

β-adrenergic blocking agents (see also in this chapter), verapamil (previously discussed).

Other rapid-acting nitrates: Isosorbide dinitrate (Sorbitrate, Isordil), erythrityl tetranitrate (Cardilate), pentaerythritol tetranitrate (P.E.T.N., Pentylan, Duotrate).

DRUGS USED IN SHOCK (THE SYMPATHOMIMETIC AMINES)

DOBUTAMINE HYDROCHLORIDE
DOBUTREY

ACTIONS

Dobutamine is a direct-acting inotropic agent whose primary site of action is on β_1 cardiac receptors, with mild activity on β_2 and α-adrenergic receptors. Hemodynamic responses to dobutamine include an increase in myocardial contractility, an increase in cardiac output, and a reduction in total peripheral resistance. Dobutamine may also increase renal perfusion. Large doses of dobutamine may increase heart rate and blood pressure.

INDICATIONS:

1. Short-term inotropic support after cardiac surgery.
2. Severe, refractory, chronic congestive heart failure.

3. Atrial fibrillation (administer digitalis prior to initiating dobutamine therapy).

CONTRAINDICATIONS:
Hypersensitivity to dobutamine. Idiopathic hypertrophic subaortic stenosis (IHSS).

PRECAUTIONS:
1. Monitor patient's blood pressure and heart rate frequently. Dobutamine may markedly increase heart rate and blood pressure, especially systolic pressure. Reduce dosage if indicated.
2. Dobutamine may increase ventricular ectopy; however, it rarely produces ventricular tachycardia.
3. Concurrent or previous use of a β blocking agent may render dobutamine ineffective.

ADVERSE REACTIONS:
Most Frequent: Increased heart rate, blood pressure, ventricular ectopic activity; nausea, headache, anginal pain, palpitations, dyspnea.

OVERDOSAGE:
Symptoms include marked changes in blood pressure or tachycardia. Treatment consists of a reduction in dosage or temporary discontinuation of the drug.

DOSAGE:
IV: 2.5 to 10 μg/kg/min.

DOPAMINE HYDROCHLORIDE
DOPASTAT, INTROPIN

ACTIONS:
Dopamine exerts its positive inotropic effect directly on cardiac β_1 receptors and indirectly by causing the release of norepinephrine from its storage sites. Dopamine is an endogenous catecholamine and a precursor of norepinephrine that has the ability to enhance cardiac output by increasing myocardial contractibility and stroke volume. An increase in renal blood flow and sodium excretion is noted owing to dopamine's ability to activate dopaminergic receptors. Large doses of dopamine stimulate α-receptor activation (which then overrides dopaminergic effects), leading to vasoconstriction, a diminished systemic vascular resistance (SVR), and correction of hypotension. Dopamine

has an onset of action within 2 to 4 minutes with a duration of less than 10 minutes.

INDICATIONS:

1. Cardiogenic shock due to myocardial infarction, trauma, septicemia, open heart surgery, renal failure, and congestive heart failure.
2. Hemodynamically significant hypotension.

CONTRAINDICATIONS:

Pheochromocytoma, tachyarrhythmias, ventricular fibrillation.

PRECAUTIONS:

1. Hypoxia, hypercapnia and acidosis may decrease dopamine's effectiveness or increase side effects. These conditions should be corrected prior to administration of dopamine.
2. Dopamine does not replace volume loss. Hypovolemia should be corrected prior to administration of dopamine.
3. Dopamine has the ability to reverse the effects of β-adrenergic blocking agents.
4. Frequent monitoring of the urine output, cardiac output, ECG and blood pressure should be done and observed for significant changes.

ADVERSE REACTIONS:

Most Frequent: Ventricular ectopy, tachycardia, anginal pain, palpitations, hypotension, vasoconstriction, dyspnea, headache, nausea and vomiting.

OVERDOSAGE:

Symptoms include a marked elevation of the blood pressure and decreased urinary output. If this occurs, reduce dosage or discontinue the drug. Since the duration of dopamine's action is short, no other measures should be necessary.

DOSAGE:

IV infusion: 2 to 5 μg/kg/min up to a rate of 20 to 50 μg/kg/min as needed for seriously ill patients. Frequent urine output checks are needed for doses in excess of 16 μg/kg/min.

ISOPROTERENOL HYDROCHLORIDE
ISUPREL

ACTIONS

Isoproterenol is a potent β-adrenergic stimulator that has the ability to stimulate the cardiac rate, rhythm, myocardial oxygen consumption, and cardiac output and to dilate resistance vessels of skeletal muscles and relax bronchial smooth muscle. It also causes reduced peripheral vascular resistance, which may cause a drop in blood pressure. Onset of action is rapid; however, duration is brief (less than 60 minutes, rapidly metabolized by COMT).

INDICATIONS:

1. Hemodynamically significant bradycardia that is refractory to atropine.
2. Bronchodilator (see Chapter 8).

CONTRAINDICATIONS:

Tachycardia caused by digitalis intoxication. Recent guidelines established by the American Heart Association state that the use of isoproterenol is contraindicated in the treatment of cardiac arrest owing to a) its possible exacerbation of ischemia and/or hypotension, b) its effects of lowering coronary perfusion pressure during cardiac arrest, and c) its effect of increasing the mortality rate as shown in experimental animal studies.

PRECAUTIONS:

1. Do not coadminister epinephrine and isoproterenol; potential adverse effects include serious arrhythmias.
2. Correct hypovolemia before administering isoproterenol.
3. Do not administer to patients with ischemic heart disease. Isoproterenol increases myocardial oxygen demand.
4. Isoproterenol may exacerbate tachyarrhythmias due to digitalis toxicity and hypokalemia.
5. Isoproterenol may reverse the effects of β-adrenergic blocking agents.

ADVERSE REACTIONS:

Cardiac: Tachycardia, palpitations.
CNS: Headache, dizziness, nervousness, tremors.
Pulmonary: Pulmonary edema, bronchial inflammation.
GI: Nausea, vomiting.

DOSAGE:

IV: 1 to 2 mg diluted in 500 ml of 5% dextrose infused at a rate of 0.5 to 5 μg/min. Adjust dosage according to heart rate response.

Other Drugs Used in Shock

Epinephrine (see Chapter 19), norepinephrine (Levophed), ephedrine (see also Chapter 8), mephentermine (Wyamine Sulfate), metaraminol (Aramine), methoxamine HCl (Vasoxyl), phenylephrine HCl (see also Chapter 7).

ANTIHYPERTENSIVE AGENTS

DIAZOXIDE
HYPERSTAT

ACTIONS:
Diazoxide is a direct-acting vasodilator that reduces blood pressure by relaxing peripheral arteriole smooth muscle. This action causes a reflex increase in heart rate and cardiac output as the blood pressure is reduced. Also, an increase in renal blood flow is noted, after an initial decrease.

INDICATIONS:
1. Hypertensive emergencies.
2. In patients with hypertensive encephalopathy, malignant hypertension (especially those associated with renal impairment), and in patients when an urgent decrease of diastolic pressure is indicated.

CONTRAINDICATIONS:
Hypersensitivity to diazoxide, compensatory hypertension.

PRECAUTIONS:
1. Since a rapid reduction in blood pressure is noted, patients must be monitored for ECG changes. Large doses have been associated with angina, myocardial infarction, cerebral infarction.
2. Repeated use may cause edema, CHF, or electrolyte imbalance (diazoxide causes sodium retention).
3. Diazoxide may cause hypotension; frequent monitoring of the blood pressure is necessary.
4. Coadministered furosemide may be used to prevent sodium and water retention. Furosemide may also enhance the antihypertensive effect of diazoxide.

ADVERSE REACTIONS:
The most common adverse reactions are hypotension, nausea and vomiting, dizziness, weakness, sodium and water retention. Larger doses (300 mg) have caused severe hypotension, angina, cerebral ischemia, hemiplegia, and myocardial infarction.

OVERDOSAGE:
To treat hypotension, place patient in the Trendelenburg position. If indicated, dopamine or epinephrine may be given to correct hypotension. Hemodialysis may be employed to remove diazoxide from the blood.

DOSAGE:

IV route only: 1 to 3 mg/kg up to a maximum of 150 mg in a single dose. May be repeated in 5- to 15-minute intervals.

NITROPRUSSIDE SODIUM
NIPRIDE

ACTIONS:

Nitroprusside is a potent direct-acting hypotensive agent that produces peripheral vasodilation of both arterial and venous vessels. In hypertensive or normotensive patients, nitroprusside causes a reduction in the arterial blood pressure, a slight increase in the heart rate, a mild decrease in cardiac output, and a reduction in total peripheral vascular resistance. In patients with left ventricular failure, nitroprusside causes an increase in cardiac output and a reduction in the pulmonary capillary wedge pressure (PCWP), in addition to its effect to cause a reduction in blood pressure. Nitroprusside has an immediate onset of action—a reduced blood pressure is noted within 30 to 60 seconds.

INDICATIONS:

1. Hypertensive emergencies.
2. For controlled hypotension during anesthesia.
3. Severe, refractory, chronic congestive heart failure.
4. Hypertensive and normotensive patients with severe, persistent pump failure associated with a low cardiac output and increased peripheral vascular resistance.

CONTRAINDICATIONS:

Treatment of compensatory hypertension (e.g., a-v shunt or coarctation of the aorta). Not indicated for use to produce or control hypotension in surgery patients with known inadequate cerebral circulation.

PRECAUTIONS:

1. Excessive doses of nitroprusside may cause cyanide toxicity. Nitroprusside is rapidly metabolized to cyanide and thiocyanate by a reaction with hemoglobin. Since metabolic acidosis is the earliest sign of cyanide toxicity, blood pH and acid-base status should be frequently monitored.
2. Use with caution in patients with hepatic and renal insufficiency.
3. Severe hypotensive effects may occur with concurrent use of other antihypertensive agents.
4. Nitroprusside may increase both myocardial and pulmonary arteriovenous shunts due to nitroprusside's action on coronary resistance vessels.

Increases in total coronary blood flow are noted, but not necessarily that portion contributing to improved perfusion.

5. Discontinue administration if blood pressure is not reduced in 10 minutes with a dose of 10 μg/kg/min.

ADVERSE REACTIONS:

Most common effects caused by a too rapid reduction in blood pressure: Nausea, retching, apprehension, palpitations, dizziness, abdominal pain, diaphoresis.

Pulmonary: May worsen the ventilation-perfusion mismatch and produce hypoxemia due to nitroprusside-induced hypotension.

OVERDOSAGE:

Discontinue infusion if profound hypotension or cyanide toxicity occurs. Symptoms of cyanide toxicity include blurred vision, headache, ataxia, dyspnea, delerium, loss of consciousness, absence of reflexes, hypotension, metabolic acidosis. Treatment consists of the administration of amyl nitrite, sodium nitrite, sodium thiosulfate. Observe patient for several hours for the possible reemergence of the signs of overdosage.

DOSAGE:

Continuous IV infusion with sterile 5% dextrose in water: 3 μg/kg/min (range 0.5 to 10 μg/kg/min).

Other Antihypertensive Agents

Diuretics: Thiazides and derivatives, indapamide, furosemide, amiloride, spironolactone.

Antiadrenergic Agents—Centrally Acting: Methyldopa (Aldomet), clonidine (Catapres), guanabenz (Wytensin).

Antiadrenergic Agents—Peripherally Acting: Reserpine (Serpalan, Serpasil), guanethidine (Ismelin Sulfate), guanadrel (Hylorel), prazosin (Minipress).

Antiadrenergic Agents—β-Adrenergic Blockers: see β-adrenergic blockers in this chapter.

Vasodilators: Hydralazine (Alazine, Apresoline), minoxidil (Loniten, Minodyl), nitroglycerin (IV) (previously discussed).

Agents For Pheochromocytoma: Phentolamine (Regitine), phenoxybenzamine (Dibenzyline), metyrosine (Demser).

Angiotensin Converting Enzyme (ACE) Inhibitors: Captopril (Capoten), enalapril maleate (Vasotec).

THE β-ADRENERGIC BLOCKING AGENTS

PROPRANOLOL HYDROCHLORIDE
INDERAL

ACTIONS:
Propranolol is the prototype β blocker. Propranolol's antiarrhythmic, antihypertensive action produces a β-adrenergic blockade on the cardiac β receptors. This effect reduces myocardial contractility, prolongs AV conduction time, and suppresses myocardial automaticity. Subsequently, this results in decreased heart rate, cardiac output, and systemic arterial pressure. Propanolol is nonselective in that it exerts its influence on both β_1- and β_2-adrenergic receptors.

INDICATIONS:
1. Dysrhythmias due to a hyperactive sympathetic nervous system.
2. Catecholamine-induced arrhythmias.
3. Supraventricular and ventricular tachyarrhythmias.
4. As a hypotensive agent in the treatment of hypertensive and anginal episodes.
5. As an adjunct with digitalis therapy to control chronic A-fib or A-flutter.
6. Myocardial infarction; to reduce cardiovascular mortality and the risk of reinfarction.

CONTRAINDICATIONS:
Severe COPD, asthma, bronchospasm. Hypersensitivity to β-adrenergic blocking agents, overt cardiac failure, sinus bradycardia, cardiogenic shock.

PRECAUTIONS:
1. Use with caution in patients with impaired renal or hepatic function.
2. The effects of succinylcholine and tubocurarine may be enhanced by adrenergic β blockers.
3. Use with caution in patients with cardiac failure; use of β_1 blockers depresses myocardial contractility and may potentiate more severe cardiac failure.
4. Use with caution in patients with hyperreactive airway disease; use of β_2 blockers may cause bronchospasm.

ADVERSE REACTIONS:
CNS: Dizziness, fatigue, vertigo, mental depression, anxiety, nervousness, behavioral changes.

Cardiovascular: Bradycardia, chest pain, angina, edema, hypotension, tachycardia, arrhythmias, palpitations, syncope, first- and third-degree heart block.
Pulmonary: Bronchospasm, dyspnea, cough, wheezes, rales, rhinitis, pharyngitis, bronchial obstruction.
GI: Nausea, vomiting, anorexia, abdominal cramping, acute pancreatitis.

OVERDOSAGE:

Treatment consists of monitoring the blood pressure and ECG. Implement respiratory support if indicated. Treat PVCs with lidocaine, hypotensive bradycardia with atropine, bronchospasm with β_2-adrenergic drug or theophylline derivative.

DOSAGE:

PO: *For arrhythmias:* Usual range—10 to 30 mg tid or qid. *For hypertension:* Usual range—120 to 240 mg per day (given bid or tid), or 120 to 160 mg once daily (sustained-release tablets). *For angina:* Usual range—160 mg per day. *For myocardial infarction:* Usual range—180 to 240 mg per day (given tid or qid). *For migraine:* Usual range—160 to 240 mg per day.
IV: 1 to 3 mg, not to exceed 1 mg/min; 2nd dose may be given after 2 minutes, thereafter, every 4 hours until desired rate and rhythm are achieved. Monitor blood pressure and ECG continuously. IV use should be reserved for life-threatening arrhythmias.

Other β-Adrenoceptor Blocking Agents

METOPROLOL
LOPRESSOR

Metoprolol is an effective antihypertensive agent that exhibits equal potency to propranolol with respect to β_1 blockade; however, metoprolol is 50- to 100-fold less potent than propranolol in blocking β_2 receptors. Metoprolol's use is advantageous in treating hypertension and myocardial infarction, especially in patients with asthma, diabetes, or peripheral vascular disease (where propranolol's β_2 action is unwanted owing to bronchoconstriction and vasoconstriction). The oral dose ranges from 100 to 450 mg/day. for prophylaxis after acute myocardial infarction, 100 mg bid.

ATENOLOL
TENORMIN

Atenolol is a long-acting β_1-selective blocker indicated for use in the treatment of angina pectoris and hypertension. Because of atenolol's cardioselectivity, it is preferred (as is metoprolol) for use in patients with asthma, diabetes, and peripheral vascular disorders. The oral dose ranges from 50 to 100 mg once daily.

LABETALOL
NORMODYNE, TRANDATE

Labetalol is a nonselective β-blocking agent (blocks both β_1 and β_2 receptors) that also exhibits postsynaptic α_1-adrenergic blocking action. Owing to labetalol's combined α and β effects, it is useful for treating hypertensive emergencies and hypertension associated with pheochromocytoma (tumor of chromaffin tissue of the adrenal medulla; the symptoms of hypertension reflect the increased production and release of epinephrine and norepinephrine). Oral dose ranges from 100 to 400 mg bid. Patients with severe hypertension may require up to 2.4 g/day. For the treatment of hypertensive emergencies: repeated (until desired blood pressure is achieved) IV bolus injections ranging from 20 to 80 mg. Full effect is usually noted after 5 minutes of the injections.

THROMBOLYTIC AGENTS

ALTEPLASE, RECOMBINANT
ACTIVASE

ACTIONS:

Alteplase is a tissue plasminogen activator (TPA) created by recombinant DNA. When introduced to the circulatory system, alteplase indirectly initiates local fibrinolysis by binding to fibrin in a thrombus and converting the entrapped plasminogen to plasmin (plasmin is a proteolytic enzyme that has a particular affinity for fibrin and the ability to dissolve formed fibrin clots).

Coronary occlusion due to a thrombus exists in the infarct-related coronary artery in the majority of patients experiencing a transmural myocardial infarction. Lysis of thrombi in the obstructed coronary vessel, reperfusion of the obstructed coronary vessel, and improved left ventricular function are noted after infusion of alteplase (treatment must be initiated as soon as possible following acute myocardial infarction symptoms).

INDICATIONS:

Alteplase is especially indicated for the destruction of thrombi in obstructed coronary vessels in the management of acute myocardial infarction (AMI).

Related effects include improved ventricular function and a reduction in the incidence of congestive heart failure.

CONTRAINDICATIONS:
Owing to the thrombolytic actions of alteplase, an increased incidence of bleeding is noted. Alteplase is contraindicated in patients with a high risk of internal bleeding, those with active internal bleeding, in patients with a history of cerebrovascular accident, and in intracranial or intraspinal surgery patients (within 2 months). Also, in patients with intracranial neoplasm, arteriovenous malformation or aneurysm, bleeding diathesis, or severe uncontrolled hypertension. Relative contraindications include major surgery, delivery of a child, organ biopsy, serious gastrointestinal bleeding, and serious trauma within the previous ten days.

PRECAUTIONS:
1. Carefully monitor patients for bleeding (especially those patients with IV sites, venous cutdowns, arterial puncture sites, etc.)
2. Arrhythmias have been noted after the infusion of alteplase (sinus bradycardia, ventricular irritability). Have antiarrhythmic therapy available.
3. Concomitant use of heparin may contribute to the incidence of bleeding. Use cautiously.
4. Spontaneous bleeding from internal sites may occur in patients with abnormal platelet count, prothrombin time, partial thromboplastin time, or bleeding time. These patients should be carefully assessed before initiating therapy.
5. Miscellaneous precautions include recent cardiopulmonary resuscitation, subacute bacterial endocarditis, mitral disease with atrial fibrillation, pregnancy, prior severe allergic reaction, advanced age (over 75).

ADVERSE REACTIONS:
The most frequent adverse reaction to alteplase therapy is bleeding, which can be subdivided into two groups: (*a*) internal bleeding (GI tract, GU tract, retroperitoneal, or intracranial sites), and (*b*) superficial or surface bleeding from various puncture sites. If serious bleeding occurs, alteplase therapy must be discontinued, as well as any concomitant anticoagulant therapy.

Other reactions include nausea, vomiting, hypotension, fever, urticaria.

DOSAGE:
Alteplase is given by IV infusion only and is initiated as soon as possible after the onset of symptoms. Recommended dose: first hour, 60 mg (34.8 million IU). 6 to 10 mg is given as a bolus within the first 1 to 2 minutes. Second hour,

20 mg (11.6 million IU). Third hour, 20 mg (11.6 million IU). An increased incidence of intracranial bleeding is noted with a dose of 150 mg. Recommended maximum dose is 100 mg given over a three-hour period.

STREPTOKINASE
KABIKINASE, STREPTASE

UROKINASE
ABBOKINASE

ACTIONS:
Urokinase directly converts plasminogen to plasmin. Plasmin then has the ability to destroy fibrin clots and fibrinogen. Streptokinase indirectly converts plasminogen to plasmin by first producing an "activator complex" (where streptokinase combines with plasminogen to produce a structural alteration in plasminogen). This active form of plasminogen is then converted to plasmin-streptokinase, from which streptokinase is detached and fragmented to form lower molecular weight products.

INDICATIONS:
Urokinase and streptokinase are the drugs of choice to treat pulmonary emboli and deep vein thrombosis in selected patients (*Ann Intern Med,* 1980). Streptokinase is also indicated in patients with acute evolving transmural myocardial infarction, arterial thrombosis and embolism, and occluded AV cannulae. Urokinase is also indicated for coronary artery thrombosis and IV catheter clearance (restores patency to IV catheters obstructed by clotted blood or fibrin).

CONTRAINDICATIONS:
Refer to alteplase.

PRECAUTIONS:
Refer to alteplase.

ADVERSE REACTIONS:
Refer to alteplase.

DOSAGE:
Streptokinase: For pulmonary embolism and deep venous thrombosis: initial loading dose of 250,000 IU given over 30 minutes, follow with 100,000 IU/hr (6 ml/hr) for 24 to 72 hours. For acute evolving transmural MI: 1,500,000 IU given over 60 minutes.

Urokinase: Initial loading dose: 2000 units/lb (4400 units/kg) as an admixture with 0.9% Sodium Chloride Injection or 5% Dextrose Injection given at a rate of 90 ml/hr over 10 minutes. Follow with 2000 units/lb/hr (4400 units/kg/hr) given at a rate of 15 ml/hr for 12 hours.

Other Anticoagulants

Heparin, warfarin sodium (Coumadin), anisindione (Miradon).

Appendices III

Assessment Test A

1. The mediators of inflammation synthesized after mast cell degranulation and collectively known as the slow-reacting substance of anaphylaxis are:

   A. The prostaglandins D_2 and $F_{2\alpha}$.
   B. The chemotactic factors NCF and ECF.
   C. The leukotrienes C_4, D_4, and E_4.
   D. Serotonin and bradykinin.

2. Mr. Salivas, a 32-year-old, 54-kg white male, has just been admitted to the emergency room with severe burn injuries and smoke inhalation following a house fire. The patient is very combative and anxious. Dr. Loren has decided to intubate for airway protection, owing to the evidence of tracheal burns and laryngeal edema. The drug of choice to induce paralysis to aid endotracheal intubation in the burn patient is:

   A. Pancuronium bromide (Pavulon)
   B. Succinylcholine chloride (Anectine)
   C. Morphine sulfate
   D. Neostigmine (Prostigmin)

3. Which of the following endogenous catecholamines participates in the synthesis of norepinephrine in the adrenergic postsynaptic effector cell?

   A. Isoetharine
   B. Epinephrine
   C. Isoproterenol
   D. Dopamine

4. Mr. Hale has just been admitted to the intensive care unit following a motor vehicle accident in which he sustained severe head injuries. Which of the following drugs would be indicated to reduce intracranial pressure and relieve cerebral edema?

   A. Furosemide (Lasix)
   B. Mannitol (Osmitrol)
   C. Acetazolamide (Diamox)
   D. Propranolol (Inderal)

5. Which of the following agents would you recommend for cholinergic-mediated bronchospasm?

   A. Albuterol
   B. Alupent
   C. Bronkosol
   D. Atropine

6. The endogenous enzyme that has the ability to inactivate the cAMP system is:

   A. Acetylcholinesterase
   B. Acetylcholine
   C. Acetyl coenzyme A
   D. Phosphodiesterase

7. Which of the following medications can be administered via inhalation as a mucokinetic agent?

   I. 0.9% NaCl
   II. Terbutaline
   III. Acetylcysteine
   IV. $NaHCO_3$
   V. Metaproterenol

   A. I, III
   B. II, III, V
   C. I, III, IV
   D. I, II, IV
   E. I, II, III, IV, V

8. Which of the following serves as the transmitter substance at the ganglionic neuroeffector junction in the sympathetic system?

A. Norepinephrine
B. Dopamine
C. Epinephrine
D. Acetylcholinesterase
E. Acetylcholine

9. Which statement(s) accurately describe competitive neuromuscular blocking agents and depolarizing neuromuscular blocking agents?

    I. Competitive blocking agents can be reversed, but depolarizing agents cannot.
    II. When a competitive blocking agent is administered, it initially causes muscle contraction.
    III. Depolarizing agents have the ability to inactivate acetylcholine receptors.
    IV. Depolarizing agents, when indicated for use, may be safely used in the burn patient.

    A. I, III
    B. II, III
    C. II, IV
    D. I, II, III
    E. III, IV

10. Which of the following have the ability to induce (either directly or indirectly) bronchodilation:

    I. The prostaglandins E_1 and E_2.
    II. β_2-Adrenergic agonists
    III. α-Adrenergic agonists
    IV. Corticosteroids
    V. Cholinergic stimulants

    A. II, IV
    B. II, IV, V
    C. I, II, IV
    D. I, II, III, IV
    E. I, II, IV, V

11. Which of the following drugs would be indicated to prevent reflex bradycardia such as that induced by oropharyngeal stimulation during intubation?

A. Inderal
B. Lidocaine
C. Atropine
D. Epinephrine

12. You are called to assess an 18-month-old patient who is exhibiting signs of respiratory distress. On examination you note a somewhat anxious child with signs of mild to moderate upper respiratory obstruction. Clinical signs and symptoms include audible respiratory stridor, a harsh barking cough, mild intercostal retractions, respirations 52 bpm, pulse 136. The chest is clear except for the respiratory stridor. You would recommend which of the following?

    A. Albuteral 0.25 ml administered via nebulizer, and cold mist tent therapy.
    B. Racemic epinephrine 0.3 ml administered via nebulizer, and cold mist tent therapy.
    C. Albuterol 0.5 ml administered via nebulizer, and cold mist tent therapy.
    D. Racemic epinephrine 1.0 ml administered via nebulizer, and cold mist tent therapy.

13. Your patient is to receive 6 ml of an 8% Mucomyst (acetylcysteine) solution to be administered via nebulization. Stock solution contains a 10% solution of Mucomyst. How much of the 10% solution of Mucomyst is needed to prepare an 8% solution?

    A. 3.2 ml
    B. 4.8 ml
    C. 6.0 ml
    D. 7.5 ml
    E. 13.3 ml

14. Referring to question 13: You have properly diluted the Mucomyst solution and are now administering it via nebulization. Five minutes into the treatment your patient becomes agitated and tachypneic. Upon auscultation, wheezes and diminished breath sounds are noted. You would:

    A. Continue the Mucomyst treatment as ordered.
    B. Dilute the Mucomyst solution further by adding more normal saline to the nebulizer.

C. Stop the treatment and inform the physician that the patient does not tolerate Mucomyst.
D. Stop the treatment and recommend to the physician that a bronchodilator be administered prior to or added with the Mucomyst treatment.

15. Which of the following are effective antifungal agents?

I. Amphotericin B
II. Kanamycin
III. Ketoconazole
IV. Ampicillin
V. Flucytosine

A. I, III, V
B. II, III, IV
C. III, V
D. I, II, IV
E. I, II, III, IV, V

16. The electrocardiogram tracing shown in Figure A.1 indicates a need for what *immediate* action?

A. The administration of epinephrine.
B. Intubation and ventilation.
C. Direct-current shock.
D. The administration of lidocaine.

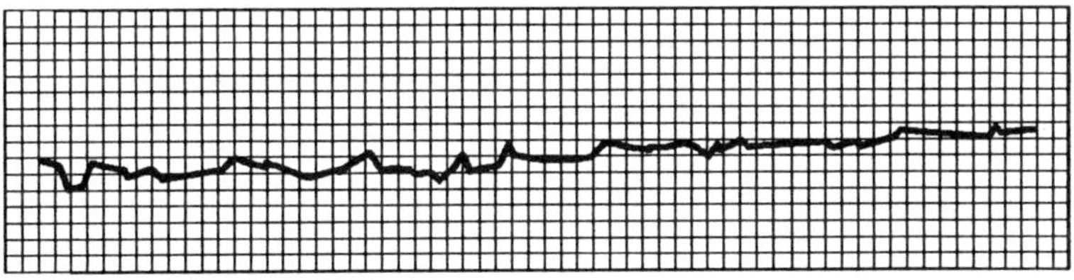

Figure A.1.

17. Which of the following drugs are indicated for myasthenia gravis?

I. Neostigmine
II. Succinylcholine
III. Edrophonium chloride
IV. Atropine
V. Pyridostigmine bromide

A. III, IV
B. I, III, V
C. II, IV
D. I, III, IV, V
E. I, II, III, IV, V

18. Which of the following medications are indicated in treating cardiac arrest?

I. Epinephrine
II. Calcium chloride
III. Lidocaine
IV. Procainamide
V. Bretylium tosylate

A. I, III
B. II, IV, V
C. III, IV, V
D. I, II, IV, V
E. I, II, III, IV, V

19. A 1:200 drug solution can also be expressed as:

A. 1.0%
B. 0.1%
C. 0.05%
D. 0.5%
E. 1 g:100 ml

20. Which of the following routes of drug administration pertain to the parenteral route?

I. Intravenous
II. Oral
III. Rectal
IV. Subcutaneous
V. Intramuscular

A. I, V
B. II, III, IV
C. IV, V
D. I, IV, V
E. I, III, IV, V

21. Which of the following drugs is the principal neurotransmitter at the postganglionic synapses of the sympathetic system?

    A. Acetylcholine
    B. Epinephrine
    C. Anticholinesterase
    D. Dopamine

22. How many milligrams of Mucomyst would your patient receive if you gave 5 ml of a 20% Mucomyst solution?

    A. 5 mg
    B. 10 mg
    C. 500 mg
    D. 1,000 mg

23. The diagnostic staining technique that determines the presence of *Mycobacterium* is:

    A. Acid-fast
    B. Gram-positive
    C. Gram-negative
    D. Culture and sensitivity

24. An intensive care unit patient is experiencing episodes of unifocal premature ventricular complexes (PVCs). You would recommend which of the following:

    A. Digitalis
    B. Defibrillation
    C. Quinidine
    D. Lidocaine

25. The agent that has the ability to convert paroxysmal supraventricular tachycardia (SVT) to sinus rhythm is:

    A. Epinephrine
    B. Streptokinase
    C. Verapamil
    D. Nitroprusside sodium

26. Which of the following is/are synthesized from arachidonic acid metabolism?

I. Histamine
II. Corticosteroids
III. Prostaglandins
IV. Leukotrienes

A. I, II, III, IV
B. I, III, IV
C. II, IV
D. II, III
E. III, IV

27. Which of the following are true statements regarding cromolyn sodium?

I. It is indicated for status asthmaticus.
II. It acts to prevent antigen-antibody reactions.
III. It is indicated for the prevention of exercise-induced bronchospasm.
IV. It is indicated as a prophylactic agent to reduce the incidence of asthmatic attacks.
V. It has the ability to prevent mast cell degranulation by blocking the influx of sodium ions entering the mast cell.

A. III, IV
B. I, III, V
C. II, V
D. III, IV, V
E. I, II, III, IV, V

28. Which of the following agents are effective in the treatment of atrial fibrillation?

I. Quinidine
II. Lidocaine
III. Epinephrine
IV. Isoproterenol
V. Digitalis

A. III only
B. I, V
C. II, IV
D. I, III, IV, V
E. I, III, V

29. Which of the following have the ability to block the β_2-adrenergic receptor?

    I. Dopamine
    II. Phentolamine
    III. α-Adrenergic agonists
    IV. Inderal
    V. Prostaglandin E series

    A. I, II
    B. III, IV, V
    C. IV only
    D. I, II, IV
    E. I, II, III, IV, V

30. Mrs. Tetros is a 68-year-old patient who has chronic obstructive pulmonary disease and a history of hypertension. Dr. Rohrer orders a regimen of atropine 1.2 mg to be alternated with albuterol 2.5 mg every 2 hours. The stock solution of atropine contains 0.4 mg/ml and the stock solution of albuterol contains 5 mg/ml. How many ml of atropine and albuterol would you give to the patient?

    A. 2 ml atropine, 0.5 ml albuterol
    B. 2 ml atropine, 1 ml albuterol
    C. 3 ml atropine, 0.5 ml albuterol
    D. 3 ml atropine, 1 ml albuterol

31. Referring to question 30: Mrs. Tetros has been receiving the atropine and albuterol regimen for 24 hours. During this time, Mrs. Tetros has developed tenacious secretions with mucus plugging. You would recommend:

    A. Continuing the present course of therapy.
    B. Deleting albuterol from Mrs. Tetros's therapy.
    C. Deleting atropine from Mrs. Tetros's therapy.
    D. Reducing the administered dose of atropine.
    E. Reducing the administered does of albuterol.

32. Mr. Gates is admitted to the hospital with acute hypertension. Which of the following drugs would best treat Mr. Gates's hypertension?

A. Dopamine
B. Digitalis
C. Isoproterenol
D. Nitroprusside

33. Mr. Simms is brought to the emergency room by the paramedics. On examination vital signs reveal blood pressure 80/54, respirations 4/min. Mr. Simms is lethargic and mildly responsive to painful stimuli. The paramedics state they found an empty bottle of codeine in his possession. Which of the following drugs will reverse the effects of codeine?

A. Doxapram (Dopram)
B. Naloxone (Narcan)
C. Morphine
D. Versed

34. The decongestants are classified as:

A. Sympathetic amines with primary α receptor actions.
B. Sympatholytics with primary α receptor antagonism.
C. Cholinergic agonists.
D. Sympathomimetics with primary β_1 effects.

35. Which of the following may be administered as a decongestant?

I. Epinephrine
II. Ephedrine
III. Phenylephrine
IV. Phenylpropanolamine

A. III only
B. I, II
C. III, IV
D. II, III, IV
E. I, II, III, IV

36. Which of the following statements are true regarding the administration of sodium bicarbonate during cardiopulmonary resuscitation?

I. Excessive administration can lead to metabolic alkalosis.
II. The use of this drug is associated with increased arterial carbon dioxide tension.

III. It has the ability to inhibit the occurrence of cardiac arrhythmias.
IV. The use of this drug improves spontaneous circulation in the compromised patient.
V. The standard dose, if given during resuscitation, is 1 mEq/kg.

A. I, II, IV
B. II, III, V
C. II, IV
D. I, II, V
E. I, II, IV, V

37. Cushing's syndrome is an adverse effect of what category of medication?

A. α-Adrenergic agonists
B. Sympathetic bronchodilators
C. Xanthines
D. Corticosteroids
E. Anticholinergics

38. The microorganism *Candida albicans* is classified in which of the following categories?

A. Protozoa
B. Fungus
C. Virus
D. Gram-negative organism
E. Anaerobic organism

39. A response that may occur with repeated and excessive use of the same drug is:

A. Potentiation
B. Synergism
C. Physical antagonism
D. Tachyphylaxis

40. The proprietary name of a drug may be described as:

A. The name given to a drug by official pharmaceutical publications.
B. The name given to a drug by the company that developed the drug.
C. The name given to a drug by the legal owner or manufacturer of the drug.
D. The drug's structural formula.

41. The drug that has the ability to block acetylcholine's action at the muscarinic receptor site through competitive inhibition is:

    A. Epinephrine
    B. Atropine
    C. Pancuronium
    D. Acetylcholinesterase

42. The optimum inhaled drug particle size for depostion *into the alveoli* is:

    A. >10 μm
    B. 10 to 5 μm
    C. 5 to 2 μm
    D. 2 to 1 μm

43. Which of the following factors may interact with the delivery of a drug to its desired site of action?

    I. Route of administration.
    II. Absorption of the drug.
    III. Distribution of the drug throughout the circulatory system.
    IV. Biotransformation of the drug.
    V. The elimination of the drug.

    A. I, III, V
    B. II, IV
    C. III, IV, V
    D. II, III, IV, V
    E. I, II, III, IV, V

44. Coadministering bronchodilators with xanthines produces an effect greater than the sum of their independent effects. This is an example of:

    A. Synergism
    B. Summation
    C. Potentiation
    D. Cummulation

45. The prototype β blocker that produces both β_1 and β_2 blockade at the adrenergic receptor site is:

    A. Isuprel
    B. Epinephrine
    C. Inderal
    D. Nipride

46. Which statement(s) accurately describe metaproterenol (Alupent)?

I. Alupent has no vasoconstricting effects.
II. Alupent has a longer duration than isoetharine (Bronkosol).
III. Alupent produces less cardiostimulation than isoproterenol (Isuprel).

A. II only
B. I, II
C. I, III
D. II, III
E. I, II, III

47. You are managing a ventilator patient in the coronary care unit following his open heart surgery. Three hours after surgery, the patient becomes extremely agitated and combative, and is setting off the high-pressure alarm of the ventilator. You would recommend:

I. Increasing the high-pressure alarm setting.
II. 20 mg IV Valium.
III. 300 mg IV doxapram.
IV. Coadministering morphine and Pavulon.

A. I, II
B. I, III
C. III only
D. IV only
E. I, IV

48. The anti-infective agent specifically indicated for respiratory syncytial virus (RSV) is:

A. Penicillin G
B. Ribavirin
C. Erythromycin
D. Pentamidine

49. True statements relative to the effects epinephrine produces include all of the following except:

A. Epinephrine increases the heart rate.
B. Epinephrine enhances myocardial contractile force and tone.
C. Epinephrine has the ability to reduce arterial blood pressure.
D. Epinephrine increases myocardial oxygen consumption.

E. Epinephrine is the drug of choice for anaphylactic shock and cardiac arrest.

50. The diuretic agent used as an adjuvant in patients with acute pulmonary edema is:

 A. Lasix
 B. Mannitol
 C. Diuril
 D. Diamox

ASSESSMENT TEST

	A	B	C	D	E		A	B	C	D	E
1.	[ ]	[ ]	[ ]	[ ]	[ ]	26.	[ ]	[ ]	[ ]	[ ]	[ ]
2.	[ ]	[ ]	[ ]	[ ]	[ ]	27.	[ ]	[ ]	[ ]	[ ]	[ ]
3.	[ ]	[ ]	[ ]	[ ]	[ ]	28.	[ ]	[ ]	[ ]	[ ]	[ ]
4.	[ ]	[ ]	[ ]	[ ]	[ ]	29.	[ ]	[ ]	[ ]	[ ]	[ ]
5.	[ ]	[ ]	[ ]	[ ]	[ ]	30.	[ ]	[ ]	[ ]	[ ]	[ ]
6.	[ ]	[ ]	[ ]	[ ]	[ ]	31.	[ ]	[ ]	[ ]	[ ]	[ ]
7.	[ ]	[ ]	[ ]	[ ]	[ ]	32.	[ ]	[ ]	[ ]	[ ]	[ ]
8.	[ ]	[ ]	[ ]	[ ]	[ ]	33.	[ ]	[ ]	[ ]	[ ]	[ ]
9.	[ ]	[ ]	[ ]	[ ]	[ ]	34.	[ ]	[ ]	[ ]	[ ]	[ ]
10.	[ ]	[ ]	[ ]	[ ]	[ ]	35.	[ ]	[ ]	[ ]	[ ]	[ ]
11.	[ ]	[ ]	[ ]	[ ]	[ ]	36.	[ ]	[ ]	[ ]	[ ]	[ ]
12.	[ ]	[ ]	[ ]	[ ]	[ ]	37.	[ ]	[ ]	[ ]	[ ]	[ ]
13.	[ ]	[ ]	[ ]	[ ]	[ ]	38.	[ ]	[ ]	[ ]	[ ]	[ ]
14.	[ ]	[ ]	[ ]	[ ]	[ ]	39.	[ ]	[ ]	[ ]	[ ]	[ ]
15.	[ ]	[ ]	[ ]	[ ]	[ ]	40.	[ ]	[ ]	[ ]	[ ]	[ ]
16.	[ ]	[ ]	[ ]	[ ]	[ ]	41.	[ ]	[ ]	[ ]	[ ]	[ ]
17.	[ ]	[ ]	[ ]	[ ]	[ ]	42.	[ ]	[ ]	[ ]	[ ]	[ ]
18.	[ ]	[ ]	[ ]	[ ]	[ ]	43.	[ ]	[ ]	[ ]	[ ]	[ ]
19.	[ ]	[ ]	[ ]	[ ]	[ ]	44.	[ ]	[ ]	[ ]	[ ]	[ ]
20.	[ ]	[ ]	[ ]	[ ]	[ ]	45.	[ ]	[ ]	[ ]	[ ]	[ ]
21.	[ ]	[ ]	[ ]	[ ]	[ ]	46.	[ ]	[ ]	[ ]	[ ]	[ ]
22.	[ ]	[ ]	[ ]	[ ]	[ ]	47.	[ ]	[ ]	[ ]	[ ]	[ ]
23.	[ ]	[ ]	[ ]	[ ]	[ ]	48.	[ ]	[ ]	[ ]	[ ]	[ ]
24.	[ ]	[ ]	[ ]	[ ]	[ ]	49.	[ ]	[ ]	[ ]	[ ]	[ ]
25.	[ ]	[ ]	[ ]	[ ]	[ ]	50.	[ ]	[ ]	[ ]	[ ]	[ ]

ANSWERS TO ASSESSMENT TEST

1. C
2. A
3. D
4. B
5. D
6. D
7. C
8. E
9. A
10. C
11. C
12. B
13. B
14. D
15. A
16. C
17. B
18. E
19. D
20. D
21. B
22. D
23. A
24. D
25. C
26. E
27. A
28. B
29. C
30. C
31. C
32. D
33. B
34. A
35. E
36. D
37. D
38. B
39. D
40. C
41. B
42. D
43. E
44. A
45. C
46. E
47. D
48. B
49. C
50. A

Approximate Dose Equivalents

B

Table B.1.
Liquid Measure[a]

Metric	Approximate Apothecary Equivalent	Metric	Approximate Apothecary Equivalent
1000 ml	1 quart	3 ml	45 minims
750 ml	1½ pints	2 ml	30 minims
500 ml	1 pint	1 ml	15 minims
250 ml	8 fluid ounces	0.75 ml	12 minims
200 ml	7 fluid ounces	0.6 ml	10 minims
100 ml	3½ fluid ounces	0.5 ml	8 minims
50 ml	1¾ fluid ounces	0.3 ml	5 minims
30 ml	1 fluid ounce	0.25 ml	4 minims
15 ml	4 fluid drams	0.2 ml	3 minims
10 ml	2½ fluid drams	0.1 ml	1½ minims
8 ml	2 fluid drams	0.06 ml	1 minim
5 ml	1¼ fluid drams	0.05 ml	¾ minim
4 ml	1 fluid dram	0.03 ml	½ minim

[a]From Dorland's illustrated medical dictionary, 27th ed. Philadelphia: WB Saunders, 1988.

Table B.2.
Weight[a]

Metric	Approximate Apothecary Equivalent	Metric	Approximate Apothecary Equivalent
30 g	1 ounce	30 mg	1/2 grain
15 g	4 drams	25 mg	3/8 grain
10 g	2 1/2 drams	20 mg	1/3 grain
7.5 g	2 drams	15 mg	1/4 grain
6 g	90 grains	12 mg	1/5 grain
5 g	75 grains	10 mg	1/6 grain
4 g	60 grains (1 dram)	8 mg	1/8 grain
3 g	45 grains	6 mg	1/10 grain
2 g	30 grains (1/2 dram)	5 mg	1/12 grain
1.5 g	22 grains	4 mg	1/15 grain
1 g	15 grains	3 mg	1/20 grain
0.75 g	12 grains	2 mg	1/30 grain
0.6 g	10 grains	1.5 mg	1/40 grain
0.5 g	7 1/2 grains	1.2 mg	1/50 grain
0.4 g	6 grains	1 mg	1/60 grain
0.3 g	5 grains	0.8 mg	1/80 grain
0.25 g	4 grains	0.6 mg	1/100 grain
0.2 g	3 grains	0.5 mg	1/120 grain
0.15 g	2 1/2 grains	0.4 mg	1/150 grain
0.12 g	2 grains	0.3 mg	1/200 grain
0.1 g	1 1/2 grains	0.25 mg	1/250 grain
75 mg	1 1/4 grains	0.2 mg	1/300 grain
60 mg	1 grain	0.15 mg	1/400 grain
50 mg	3/4 grain	0.12 mg	1/500 grain
40 mg	2/3 grain	0.1 mg	1/600 grain

[a]From Dorland's illustrated medical dictionary, 27th ed. Philadelphia: WB Saunders, 1988.

ORPHAN DRUGS C

Information on rare diseases and orphan drugs is supplied by the National Information Center for Orphan Drugs and Rare Diseases (NICODARD). An orphan drug is one that is useful for the diagnosis, treatment, or prevention of a rare disease or condition. A rare disease is identified as one that affects fewer than 200,000 persons in the United States or one in which expected drug sales will not cover the cost of developing and making the drug available for use. The following list includes some of the drugs and biologicals which have received orphan status.

Drug (Trade Name)	Proposed Use
Aconiazide	Treatment of tuberculosis
α_1-Antitrypsin (recombinant DNA origin)	α_1-Antitrypsin deficiency in the zz phenotype population
α_1-Proteinase inhibitor	α_1 P1 congenital deficiency
Amsacrine (Amsidyl)	Acute adult leukemia
Anagrelide	Polycythemia vera, essential thrombocytopenia
Antimelanoma antibody (XMMME-001-RTA)	Stage III melanoma not suitable to surgery
Antithrombin III	Hereditary AT-III deficiency
Antithrombin III (human) (AT-III) (Antithrombin)	
Antithrombin III (AT-III)	
AS-101	Treatment of AIDS
Bacitracin (Altracin)	Antibiotic-associated pseudomembranous enterocolitis

Drug (Trade Name)	Proposed Use
Bethanidine	Treatment of primary ventricular fibrillation
BW 12C	Treatment of sickle cell disease crisis
Colchicine	Arrest progression of neurologic disability caused by chronic progressive multiple sclerosis
Copalymer 1 (COP1)	Treatment of multiple sclerosis
Cromolyn sodium (Cromoral, Gastrocrom)	Mastocytosis Vernal keratoconjunctivitis
Cyproterone acetate (Cyproteron/Androcur)	Severe hirsutism
Dextran sulfate sodium	Treatment of AIDS
Diaziquone	Primary brain malignancies (Grade III-IV astrocytomas)
2′,3′-Dideoxyadenosine	Treatment of AIDS
Diethyldithiocarbamate (Imuthiol)	Treatment of AIDS
Digoxin antibody Sheep antidigoxin Fab (Digidote)	Life-threatening acute cardiac glycoside (digitalis) intoxication
2,3-Dimercaptosuccinic acid (DMSA)	Lead poisoning in children
Dipalmitoyl-phosphatidylcholine (DPPC)/phosphatidylglycerol (PG)—ALEC (Artificial Lung Expanding compound)	Prevention and treatment of neonatal respiratory distress syndrome (RDS)
Eflornithine HCl	Treatment of *Pneumocystis carinii* pneumonia in AIDS patients; *Trypanosoma brucei gambiense* sleeping sickness
Epoprostenol (prostacyclin, PGI_2, PGX) (Flolan) (Cyclo-Prostin)	Replacement of heparin in some hemodialysis patients
Erwinia L-Asparaginase	Acute lymphoblastic leukemia
Ethanolamine oleate	Bleeding esophageal varices
Factor XIII (Fibrogammin)	Congenital Factor XIII deficiency
Flumecinol (Zixoryn)	Hyperbilirubinemia in neonates unresponsive to phototherapy
Hexamethylmelamine (Hexastat)	Advanced ovarian adenocarcinoma
HPA-23	Treatment of AIDS
Hydroxycobalamin/sodium thiosulfate	Treatment of severe acute cyanide poisoning
Interferon alfa-nl (Wellferon)	Treatment of Kaposi's sarcoma in AIDS patients
levo-alpha-acetylmethadol or LAAM	Treatment of heroin addiction

Drug (Trade Name)	Proposed Use
Midodrine HCl	Idiopathic orthostatic hypotension
Monoclonal antibodies (murine or human) recognizing B-cell lymphoma idiotypes	B-cell lymphoma
Monoclonal antiendotoxin antibody (XMMEN-OES)	Treatment of Gram-negative sepsis that has progressed to shock
PEG-adenosine deaminase or PEG-ADA (Imudon)	Enzyme replacement for ADA deficiency in patients with severe combined immunodeficiency (SCID)
Piritrexim isethionate	Treatment of infections caused by *Pneumocystis carinii, Toxoplasma gondii,* and *Mycobacterium avium-intracellulare*
Polyribonucleotide (Anpligen)	Treatment of AIDS
Prednimustine	Malignant non-Hodgkin's lymphomas
Pulmonary surfactant	Prevention and treatment of respiratory distress syndrome (RDS)
Quinacrine HCl	Prevention of the recurrence of pneumothorax in high-risk patients (e.g., cystic fibrosis)
Selegiline HCl (Deprenyl)	Adjuvant in parkinsonism
Sodium γ-hydroxybutyrate or GHB	Narcolepsy and auxiliary symptoms of cataplexy, sleep paralysis, hypnagogic hallucinations, and automatic behavior
Sodium tetradecyl sulfate (Sotradecol)	Bleeding esophageal varices
*d,*l-Sotalol HCl	Prevention and treatment of life-threatening tachyarrhythmias
Spiramycin (Rovamycine)	Symptomatic relief and parasitic cure of chronic cryptosporidiosis in immunodeficient patients
Surface active extract of saline lavage of bovine lungs (Infasurf)	Prevention and treatment of respiratory failure due to pulmonary surfactant deficiency in preterm infants
Surfactant (human) (amniotic fluid derived)	Prevention and treatment of neonatal respiratory distress syndrome (RDS)
Teniposide or VM-26	Refractory childhood acute lymphocytic leukemia (ALL)
Thyrotropin-releasing hormone	Amyotrophic lateral sclerosis (ALS)
Trimetrexate gluconate	Treatment of *Pneumocystis carinii* pneumonia in AIDS patients
Viloxazine HCl (Vivalan)	Narcolepsy and cataplexy

Bibliography D

Albanese J, Bond T. Drug interactions: basic principles and clinical problems. New York: McGraw-Hill, 1978.

AMA Division of Drugs. AMA drug evaluations. 6th ed. Philadelphia: WB Saunders, 1986.

Anthony C, Thibodeau G. Textbook of anatomy and physiology. 11th ed. St. Louis: CV Mosby, 1983.

Ariens EJ, Simonis AM. Drug action: target tissue, dose-response relationships, and receptors. In: Teorell T, Dedrick RL, Condliffe PG. Pharmacology and pharmacokinetics. New York: Plenum Press, 1974.

Billups N, Billups S. American Drug Index. 35th ed. Philadelphia: JB Lippincott, 1991.

Burton G, Hodgkin J. Respiratory care: a guide to clinical practice. 3rd ed. Philadelphia: JB Lippincott, 1991.

Byron P, Phillips E, Kuhn R. Ribavirin administration by inhalation: aerosol-generation factors controlling drug delivery to the lung. Respir Care 1988;33:1011.

Chernow B, Lake C. The pharmacologic approach to the critically ill patient. Baltimore: Williams & Wilkins, 1988.

Clark W, Brater D, Johnson A. Goth's medical pharmacology. 12th ed. St. Louis: CV Mosby, 1988.

Conte J, Barriere S. Manual of antibiotics and infectious diseases. 6th ed. Philadelphia: Lea & Febiger, 1988.

Corkery K, Luce J, Montgomery B. Aerosolized pentamidine for treatment and prophylaxis of *Pneumocystis carinii:* an update. Respir Care 1988;33:676.

Darin J. The mode of action of cyclic AMP. Respir Care 1981;26:228.

Drug facts and comparisons. St. Louis: Facts and Comparisons, 1990.

Drug interactions and side effects index. 45th ed. Montvale, NJ: Medical Economics, 1991.

Edmunds M. Nursing drug reference: a practitioner's guide. Bowie, MD: Brady Communications, 1985.

Goodman L, Gilman A. The Pharmacological basis of therapeutics. 8th ed. New York: Macmillan, 1990.

Govoni L, Hayes J. Drugs and nursing implications. 6th ed. Norwalk, CT: Appleton and Lange, 1988.

Harkness R. Drug interactions handbook. Englewood Cliffs, NJ: Prentice-Hall, 1984.
Hayes AH Jr. How drugs affect drugs. Emerg Med 1981;13:114.
Hökfelt T, Lundberg JM, Schultzberg M, et al. Cellular localization of peptides in neural structures. Proc R Soc Lond [Biol]. 1980;210:63.
Iversen L. Amino acids and peptides: fast and slow chemical signals in the nervous system? (The Ferrier Lecture, 1983). Proc R Soc Lond [Biol]. 1984;221:245.
Julien R. A primer of drug action. 5th ed. Salt Lake City: WH Freeman, 1988.
Katzung B. Basic and clinical pharmacology. 3rd ed. Norwalk, CT: Appleton and Lange, 1987.
Kersten L. Comprehensive respiratory nursing. Philadelphia: WB Saunders, 1989.
Knoben J, Anderson P. Handbook of clinical drug data. 6th ed. Hamilton, IL: Drug Intelligence Publications, 1988.
Mathewson HS. Drugs for prevention of sudden death. Respir Care 1982;27:1536.
McPherson S. Respiratory therapy equipment. 4th ed. St. Louis: CV Mosby, 1990.
National Institutes of Health Consensus Development Conference. Thrombolytic therapy in thrombosis. Ann Intern Med 1980;93:141.
Nunn J. Applied respiratory physiology. 3rd ed. London: Butterworths, 1987.
Nursing 91 drug handbook. Springhouse, PA: Springhouse, 1991.
Nursing now: drug interactions. Springhouse, PA: Springhouse, 1984.
Physician's desk reference. 45th ed. Montvale, NJ: Medical Economics, 1991.
Pratt R, Osol A (eds). United States dispensatory and physician's pharmacology. Philadelphia: JB Lippincott.
Pratt W, Fekety R. The antimicrobial drugs. New York: Oxford University Press, 1986.
Rau J. Respiratory care pharmacology. 3rd ed. Chicago: Year Book, 1989.
Rizack M, Hillman C. Handbook of adverse drug interactions. New York: The Medical Letter, 1985.
Shapiro B, Harrison R, Trout C. Clinical application of respiratory care. 4th ed. Chicago: Year Book, 1989.
Smoker J, Tangen M, Ferree S, Hess D, Rexrode W. A protocol to assess and administer aerosol bronchodilator therapy. Respir Care 1986;31:780.
Spratto G, Loebl S. The nurse's drug handbook. 4th ed. New York: Wiley, 1986.
Temple D. Drugs affecting the respiratory system. Washington, DC: American Chemical Society, 1980.
Teplitz L. Clinical close-up on atropine. Nursing 89 1989;19(11):44.
United States pharmacopeia. National formulary. Rockville, MD: United States Pharmacopeial Convention, 1989.
Wilson D, Wilson W. Human anatomy. 2nd ed. New York: Oxford University Press, 1983.
Ziment I. Respiratory pharmacology and therapeutics. Philadelphia: WB Saunders, 1978.

INDEX

Page numbers in *italics* denote figures; those followed by "t" denote tables.